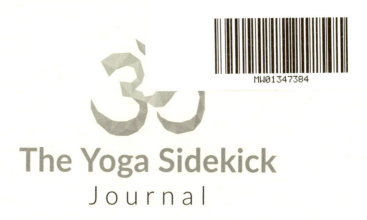

The Yoga Sidekick Journal

VOLUME 1

Flow Your Way
To Good Health.

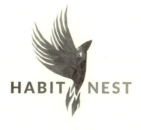

Your home for building healthy lifestyle habits.

habitnest.com

Copyright ©2022 Every Damn Day, LLC
All rights reserved.
Published by Every Damn Day, LLC.

No part of this publication may be reproduced, or stored in a retrieval system, or transmitted in any form or by any means, electronic, mechanical, recording, photocopying, scanning or otherwise, without express written permission of the publisher.

For information about permission to reproduce elections from this book,
email **team@habitnest.com**

Visit our website at **habitnest.com**

Publishers Disclaimer

While the publisher and author have used their best efforts in preparing this book, they make no representations or warranties with respect to the accuracy or completeness of the contents of this book. The advice and strategies contained herein may not be suitable for your situation. You should consult with a professional where appropriate. Neither the publisher nor the author shall be liable for any loss of profit or any other commercial damages, including but not limited to special, incidental, consequential, or other damages. The company, product, and service names used in this book are for identification purposes only. All trademarks and registered trademarks are the property of their respective owners.

Special Thanks

We'd like to extend a wholehearted, sincere thank you to the Habit Nest team for all their help in bringing this project to life. Learn more about us here: **habitnest.com/pages/about-us**

We love ya!

Exercises Disclaimer

The exercises provided by Habit Nest™ (and habitnest.com) are meant to serve as a general guide and are not to be interpreted as a recommendation for a specific treatment plan, product, or course of action. The exercises provided are not without their risks, and this or any other exercise program may result in injury. They include, but are not limited to: risk of injury, aggravation of a pre-existing condition, or adverse effect of over-exertion such as muscle strain, abnormal blood pressure, fainting, disorders of heartbeat, and very rare instances of heart attack. To reduce the risk of injury, before beginning this or any exercise program, please consult a healthcare provider for appropriate exercise prescription and safety precautions. While this is an exercise guide, it is not intended to be a direct fit for each person. It is imperative that each person tweaks the program to work for them in a way that suits their personal needs best, especially from a safety standpoint. Do not perform any exercises that cause you pain in any way. Consult with a certified personal trainer to help guide you through each exercise in person to assure they are all being done properly and in ways that will minimize injury.

The exercise instruction and advice presented are in no way intended as a substitute for medical consultation. Habit Nest™ disclaims any liability from and in connection with this program. As with any exercise program, if at any point during your workout you begin to feel faint, dizzy, or have physical discomfort, you should stop immediately and consult a physician.

Information Disclaimer

The information provided by Habit Nest™ (and habitnest.com) is for educational and entertainment purposes only, and is not to be interpreted as a recommendation for a specific treatment plan, product, or course of action. Habit Nest™ does not provide specific medical advice, and is not engaged in providing medical services. Habit Nest™ does not replace consultation with a qualified health or medical professional who sees you in person, for the health and medical needs of yourself or a loved one. In addition, while Habit Nest™ frequently updates its contents, medical, health and fitness information changes rapidly, and therefore, some information may be out of date. Please see a physician or health professional immediately if you suspect you may be ill or injured. Before implementing any nutritional information provided, consult with a nutritionist as well to make sure you can fit your personal health and nutrition needs.

ISBN: 9781950045259   First edition

The Habit Nest Mission

We are a team of people obsessed with taking ACTION and learning new things as quickly as possible.

We love finding the fastest, most effective ways to build a new skill, then systemizing that process for others.

With building new habits, we empathize with others every step of the way because we go through the same process ourselves. We live and breathe everything in our company.

We use our hard-earned intuition to outline beautifully designed, intuitive products to help people live happier, more fulfilled lives.

Everything we create comes with a mix of bite-sized information, strategy, and accountability. This hands you a simple yet drastically effective roadmap to build any skill or habit with.

We take this a step further by diving into published scientific studies, the opinions of subject-matter experts, and the feedback we get from customers to further enhance all the products we create.

Ultimately, Habit Nest is a practical, action-oriented startup aimed at helping others take back decisional authority over every action they take. We're here to help people live wholesome, rewarding lives at the brink of their potential!

– Amir Atighehchi, Ari Banayan, & Mikey Ahdoot. Cofounders of Habit Nest

Contents

Page

9 The Why
- Understanding Your Why

13 The Who
- The Three Factors of Behavior Change
- Establishing Your Identity
- Holding Yourself Accountable

19 The What
- What Is Yoga?
- The Body-Breath Connection
- Perfectionists, Tread Lightly

27 The How
- What You'll Need
- Choosing a Time & Place
- Before You Get Started

33 Let's Get Started!
- What to Expect
- The Daily Content
- One Simple Idea
- Commit

Page

40 Phase 1 (Flow 01-07)

72 Phase 2 (Flow 08-21)

132 Phase 3 (Flow 22-66)

317 Fin

- So... What Now?
- Meet the Habit Nest Team
- Shop Habit Nest Products
- What Habit Will You Conquer Next?
- Share the Love

Our Mission in Creating This Journal

Sometimes, it isn't easy to motivate yourself to exercise, or to calm your mind and remain relaxed during stressful situations.

Developing an authentic yoga practice - one that's deeply rooted in its ancient Indian origins despite being heavily westernized - can help.

Our goal in creating this journal was to make it as easy as possible for you to develop a meaningful yoga practice, get moving, and stick to your yoga goals. Along the way, you'll get all of the motivation, inspiration, and information necessary to deepen your practice.

The goal here is to present you with a decolonized and easily understandable view of each important aspect of yoga, while stoking the flames of your motivation and holding you accountable to reaching the goals you've set for yourself.

Have an amazing workout, watch incredibly fast progress happen right before your eyes, and ultimately feel supremely confident in your body.

We created this all-in-one yoga teacher & tracker so that you don't have do ANY thinking when it comes to your daily yoga practice.

If you can make the commitment to get into exercise mode, open the book, and start the first flow, you'll find yourself pushing harder than ever before without even realizing how it happened.

We created this journal to help you actually achieve your wellbeing and fitness goals.

The Why

Understanding Your Why

As humans, what sets us apart from other animals is our desire to be great as opposed to simply surviving. We all have a vision of what our ideal life might look like.

The absolute most important aspect of changing your life for the better is... **Knowing your damn Why.**

The thing is, when we forget (and we forget quite often) the reason we're struggling to improve any given aspect of our lives, we tend to retreat to our habitual selves - to the person we were before we made the decision to change.

Having a clear understanding of your 'why' (what you want to change and why you want to change it) is what pulls you through the tough times you will inevitably face when altering your habits.

Here are a few simple questions that you should take your time to sincerely answer before moving on.

The point of this is to get to the root of what drove you to embark on this new journey with of building a yoga practice.

If you're going to even make an attempt at this, you better know why you're doing it in the first place.

Seriously. Take the time to define your dream life.

BEFORE

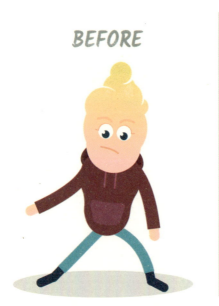

AFTER YOUR WHY

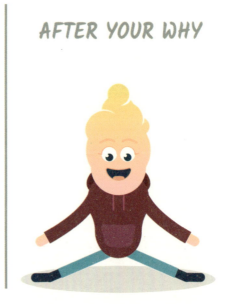

1. What will my life look like if I prioritize this habit for the next 30 days? What benefits or improvements do I hope to see?

2. What sort of ripple effect would practicing yoga have on other areas of my life? On other people's lives around me?

3. What will my life look like if I don't develop this habit? How might my mental and physical well-being be affected if I don't stick with it?

4. What goals (whether big or small) do I hope to achieve by developing a yoga practice? How exactly will developing this habit align me with those goals?

Bonus Question: What obstacles, if any, do I anticipate running into? How might I overcome them?

Bookmark this section and flip back here the next time you're struggling to stay consistent with this habit.

This section is your SOS Lifeline.

The Who

The Three Factors of Behavior Change

James Clear, author of *Atomic Habits*, writes that there are essentially three parts to behavior change (we love your work, James!).

1. The Outcomes

The **first** is the outside layer: The Outcomes. This is synonymous with your goals. An example of setting your outcomes is:

> "I want to develop a consistent yoga practice."

Outcomes are most useful at setting a larger, over-arching vision for where you want to go. The downsides of over-focusing on your outcomes are relying on hitting your goals to bring you happiness instead of enjoying the process, and a lack of practicality for what to do day-to-day.

Your outcomes are likely to change over the course of your life to match your ever-evolving goals and needs.

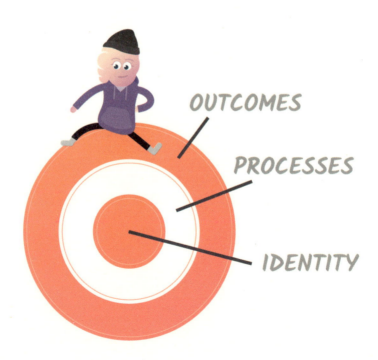

2. The Processes

The **second**, middle layer, is about processes — this boils down to what system and action steps you put in place to allow your outcomes to come to fruition. These are things like:

> *"I will practice yoga for at least ten minutes daily this week,"* or
> *"I will find poses that pinpoint my problem areas."*

This is synonymous with strategies and tactics. These can be very useful, especially when you find one that clicks, and you'll see a number for you to experiment with, sprinkled throughout the journal.

These processes are likely to change over time as you test them out. See what works best for you and switch things up when you get bored / desensitized to them.

3a. Your Identity

This one's the **big kahuna**. This is the inner-most layer, identifying what your internal belief is of yourself as a person. The biggest mistake people make in enacting behavior change is placing way too large of a focus on the first two parts of this puzzle, while entirely forgetting about the third and the most impactful — how you view yourself.

By properly emphasizing WHO you want to grow into, you will maximize your self-respect, satisfaction, and ability to control your actions — more than any motivation or strategy can give you. Use this to guide you over time.

An example of setting your identity is:

> *"I choose to practice yoga every day because I'm the type of person who takes care of my body, and I know it's important."*

After defining the identity you want to grow into for yourself, chances are this will **not change much**, but rather, only **strengthen over time** based on your actions.

3b. Your Identity on Your Off-Days

As much as this plays a role in building towards your goals, *it's equally as important in regard to times when you fall off the wagon*.

Most people subconsciously forget about what their self-identity looks like when this happens, allowing a massive negative self-view to kick in.

This leads to a major emotional factor, **guilt**, to kick in, and as many studies have shown, **guilt is a willpower destroyer**.

Instead, mindfully set your identity in these situations...

Grow into the person who uses every opportunity of falling off-track to further strengthen your ability to **switch from your off-days back to getting on track.**

Chances are, you won't be able to squeeze in a full yoga flow every single day for the rest of your life, right? Life is about knowing which habits to employ, at the right time, to help you get the most fulfillment out of life.

This involves testing different things and seeing how they serve your life's purpose. In order to really do this, you must master the ability to switch back and forth and discover how to quickly rebuild the momentum you had with your habits, without any guilt that you 'lost your mojo.'

Be the type of person who can forgive themselves for mistakes, who will love themselves unconditionally, and who can be their own best friend (because if you can't, who will?).

We know these are big emphases on emotional states that can come off as 'fluffy,' but the truth is, our fulfillment in life directly ties to our emotional states. Learning how to master them is the true feat of this journal, not just building up a specific habit.

Establishing Your Identity

Write your identity statement here.

What kind of person do you want to grow into through this process?

What kind of person do you want to be when you fall off the wagon of your habits? What do you want to remember about who you are, and how can you repurpose these days to serve your life?

Holding Yourself Accountable

Accountability is yet another vital element in creating and sticking to new habits. You can hold yourself accountable and make sure you stay consistent with your yoga practice by:

- **Finding an accountability partner.** It could be someone that's equally as committed to developing a yoga practice as you, or just someone who checks in with you to ensure you've completed your routine that day.

- **Having reasonable standards for yourself.** Start small, take your time, and don't beat yourself up for shortening your session or modifying difficult poses. *Yoga isn't about doing impressive poses*, it's about meeting and accepting yourself wherever you are in that moment.

- **Prioritizing consistency over perfection.** If you're having an off day or struggling to find motivation, it's much better to do a shortened/imperfect yoga session than to not do it at all! That consistency is the key to turning your practice into an actual habit.

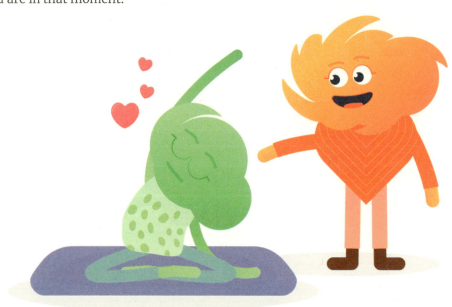

The What

What Is Yoga?

The ancient practice of yoga has roots that stretch at least as far back as 5,000 years ago, originating in Egypt and the Indus Valley. The word yoga itself means a bringing-together or unification, presumably between the mind and body.

While yoga often brings to mind the workout aspect commonly seen in Western culture, yoga is actually much more than just a form of exercise — it's a lifestyle that encompasses whole-body health, well-being, and mindset.

Yoga can be practiced through a variety of activities, but breathwork, meditation, and exercise/movement are the most common.

The Eight Limbs of Yoga

To better understand the full scope of yoga as a lifestyle, it helps to take a look at the Eight Limbs of Yoga:

- **Yamas** - A set of 5 ethical/behavioral standards surrounding how we conduct ourselves.
- **Niyamas** - A set of 5 standards regarding self-discipline and spiritual growth.
- **Asanas** - The physical poses and movements used in yoga exercise flows.
- **Pranayama** - Tuning in to & controlling your breath through various techniques and exercises.
- **Pratyahara** - The practice of withdrawing from external sensory stimuli to seek inner awareness, growth, and spiritual transcendence.
- **Dharana** - The skill of concentration and being able to focus on the task at hand.
- **Dhyana** - Developing the skill and consistent practice of meditation.
- **Samadhi** - The final limb (step) in one's spiritual journey, otherwise referred to as enlightenment.

These eight limbs were originally outlined in the Yoga Sutras (scriptures) by a sage known only as Patañjali around 500 B.C. They have since been studied extensively by scholars in various fields, as well as adapted as a core framework of Yoga by practitioners worldwide.

Throughout your journey, we'll guide you through exploring, understanding, and applying each of these limbs — in your practice, and in your life!

Main Forms of Yoga

Modern Yoga forms that focus primarily on the physical aspects fall under the umbrella of Hatha Yoga, but Hatha encompasses several more-specific practice forms that we'll be including in your daily flows.

We've included elements from each of the Hatha styles below to ensure you build a balanced and beneficial yoga practice!

- **Vinyasa** - This is the main focus of our yoga flows. Vinyasa is all about synchronizing the flow of your breaths with the flow of your body.

- **Iyengar** - Iyengar focuses heavily on alignment and holding postures, often using multiple props. Poses are held for extended periods of time so you can slowly ease yourself deeper into the pose.

- **Ashtanga** - Although it's very similar to Vinyasa yoga, Ashtanga is typically more intense. This form heavily emphasizes the lifestyle and behavioral principles of the Eight Limbs of Yoga.

- **Yin** - This is a much more meditative form of yoga that involves holding seated poses for extended periods of time. It's especially helpful for finding internal peace and external relaxation.

- **Kundalini** - This style involves a balanced mix of both physical and spiritual. It focuses on releasing Kundalini energy, which is said to be coiled around the spine. Sessions are fast-paced and often involve chanting and meditation.

- **Restorative** - Restorative Yoga is all about relaxing, healing, and winding down your mind and body. Many poses are modified to be easier and more comfortable.

Benefits of a Comprehensive Yoga Practice

Going beyond just the physical exercise aspect of yoga, a comprehensive practice can be beneficial in a multitude of ways:

- Yoga can improve ***strength, balance, and flexibility***
- A consistent yoga practice ***tones the muscles***
- Practicing yoga early in the day can help ***promote good sleep*** at bedtime
- Many of the movements and stretches help to ***relieve muscle pain*** and ***injuries***

- The physical activity and breathwork involved in yoga serve to **greatly improve** circulation, respiratory health, and digestive system regulation
- Studies suggest that yoga helps **boost the immune system**
- Yoga is shown to decrease stress and **improve** symptoms of **depression and anxiety**

Key Terms You'll See

We strive to be respectful of the culture that yoga comes from, so we will also explore the ancient teachings in-depth to ensure that you'll experience yoga as far more than just a workout.

Here are the yoga terms you'll encounter (and learn much more about!) along the way:

- **Yogi** - Anyone who consistently practices yoga.
- **Namaste** - A traditional greeting that translates to "the divine in me sees the divine in you."

  This is expressed by placing the palms together in front of the heart and is often said by yoga teachers and students at the end of each class.

- **Savasana** - This refers to a specific pose called *Corpse Pose*, which is included at the end of each flow and is commonly used to close out a yoga session.

  This pose simply involves lying supine on the floor with your eyes closed, in a meditative state.

- **Chakras** - 7 energy points that run from the top of your head to the base of your spine. Yoga is said to help align and unblock our Chakras!

- **Koshas** - We are all said to have 5 layers (or sheaths) of existence that can be strengthened and balanced by developing a comprehensive yoga practice.

- **Doshas** - According to the Ancient Indian healing science of Ayurveda, there are 3 Doshas (or bodily energy centers) derived from the 5 elements *(fire, water, earth, air, and ether)*. Everyone is said to have a dominant Dosha (or combination), and supporting the Doshas through yoga is said to create a healthy mind-body balance.

The Body-Breath Connection

Breath control is a key aspect of yoga, especially when flowing through a sequence of poses. It's also an important element of achieving a meditative state. As you go through your yoga routine, try to keep your breaths deep, slow, and synchronized with your movements.

With or without yoga, breathwork is extremely beneficial for your body. Studies show that consistent breathwork:

- Trains our brains to have sharper focus and concentration
- Can help us to reduce (or at least better cope with) chronic pain or discomfort
- Quickly reduces stress & anxiety
- Better oxygenates your body and improves circulation
- Lowers blood pressure

Building breath control requires mindfulness and awareness of your breath through various techniques and exercises. You'll encounter some new techniques and exercises along the way that will help you develop a connection between breath and movement.

If you start to get your movements and breaths out of sync, try to remember this general rule of thumb:

- **Inhale** during movements that involve *opening, stretching, or expanding* your body (e.g. stretching out your limbs, or opening up the chest)
- **Exhale** for movements that involve *making your body smaller or contracting inward* (e.g. drawing limbs in closer to the body, curling inward/forward folds, or releasing stretches).

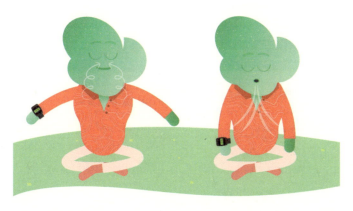

Perfectionists, Tread Lightly

The Importance of Not Getting Caught Up With Being 'Perfect.'

We include this section in 'The How' because how you actually build a new habit is heavily dependent on staying consistent with it, which itself is heavily dependent on how doing it makes you feel, which is further heavily dependent on being okay with not being perfect.

Of course, ideally, we'll stick with our scheduled yoga practice every day and absolutely crush our wellbeing goals. It doesn't seem so difficult, right?

Wrong. Besides simply forgetting about our goal, there will be times that you think about the goal and still fail to make time for your practice, or something will come up that derails your plans for the day.

This is ALL part of the process, and the more you're okay with being imperfect, the longer you'll stick to this, and the more it'll benefit you.

There's a problem with shooting for perfection from the very start.

Shooting for perfection can prevent you from ever taking one step in the direction of your goal.

So often you see people getting caught up in finding the best way to start working out, the best diet to lose weight, the most up-to-date research on the amount of sleep you need to be getting to feel amazing throughout the day... but we'll let you in on a little secret.

There's one simple concept that shatters all the best research, tips and strategies you can look for (that you'll be getting through this journal).

Here it is... the best way to crush your wellbeing goals through yoga...

You start doing SOMETHING.

You start taking SOME actions towards your goal.

You make SOME effort.

Don't waste your energy fantasizing and searching. The best way to start this process is by taking ONE step forward.

Don't let the desire to reach perfection prevent you from sticking to and growing your personal yoga practice!

Not only is perfection unattainable, but the end goal of yoga negates the idea of perfection. It's about reaching a state of *being* instead of *doing,* a state in which you separate yourself from the constant focus on outcomes and tune in to the present.

Your practice will never be perfect.

It will involve plenty of experimentation, tweaking, and personalization to make it uniquely suited to YOU.

This is your practice. There's no need to compare it to anyone else's practices, standards, or ideals. You'll be getting all the information and motivation you need from us on a daily basis in the form of daily content.

You won't PERSONALLY think every piece of content is useful. You won't think every tip will be effective. You won't think every podcast is insightful. You won't think every affirmation is worthwhile.

But if you make an attempt to use every piece of content, you'll see results. Pinky promise. Disregard the upside you expect out of it before trying it — take action first.

Every little action you take propels a snowball effect that greatly impacts other areas of your life.

Success is all about taking small, consistent actions over time.

In fact, practically every single person who has tried to build and maintain a habit has failed to follow it at some point.

Instead of trying to gloss over this, we're choosing to take a more practical approach by preparing specifically for those days of failure that will most likely blindside you when you least expect it (e.g. when your motivation is high, or something sneaks up on you).

There are two keys to using these struggle days in a way that will benefit you:

First, empathize with yourself in that situation. Don't just think about it, actually feel what you'd be experiencing (e.g. if you were very motivated one day, but you slipped up the next). Put yourself in that headspace.

Second, write out what the most disciplined version of yourself would do in that state, post-failure.

Some examples of what your most disciplined self might do:

- Remove all guilt as you realize it's useless. Instead, you immediately search for WHY this happened.

- Get genuinely excited to keep going because you realize that you love challenges - each one you surpass makes you a stronger person.

- Understand that, this time, you're mentally equipped with all you need to avoid repeating this mistake in the future.

- Acknowledge that this is a completely normal part of the self-improvement process - you gather all your energy, recoup mentally, and attack your goals, regardless.

Now, for the first time you truly struggle – what would you tell yourself and what would your actions be?

....
....
....
....
....
....
....
....

You don't have to do this exactly when you face your first struggle point, but having this as a reference can be extremely useful.

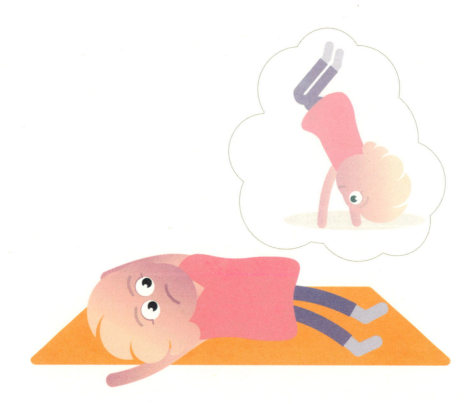

The How

What You'll Need

- **What to wear** - Much as you would for any other workout, you'll want to wear something that's comfortable and allows for full mobility/range of motion. Avoid wearing anything that's too tight, baggy, cold/warm, or distracting. Short-sleeved shirts, tank tops, sports bras, leggings, and joggers are all great options!

- **Yoga mats** - Having a yoga mat isn't absolutely required, but it definitely helps! Mats can help define the space necessary for performing each pose, provide a comfortable level of cushioning, and prevent accidental slipping.

If you don't have a mat, no worries! Standing poses can easily be done without a mat, and you can use a blanket or thick towel underneath you for poses that require you to lie down or come down onto the floor.

Props: Optional, But Helpful

Yoga can be practiced anywhere, at any time, by anyone! However, some items (props) can truly help to enhance your yoga practice.

Props are completely optional, but they can be used to help us achieve deeper stretches, modify difficult poses, or simply get into and hold poses more comfortably.

The most common props are:

- **Straps** - allow you to reach deeper stretches, and are great for anyone struggling with or working on improving their flexibility. They're typically adjustable so that you can lengthen or shorten the strap depending on the pose, your comfort, and your ability.

    (Note: If you don't have a strap, a towel works as an alternative!)

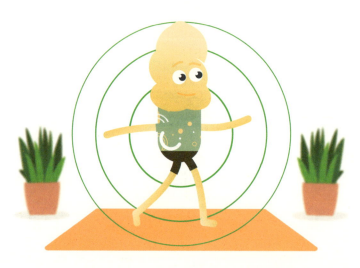

- **Blocks** - allow for reaching otherwise difficult poses, deepening stretches, or staying supported in poses that require a lot of balance or stability. They can even be used to increase the intensity and make poses more challenging.

  For example, placing blocks under your hands for Downward Facing Dog makes the pose easier, while placing the blocks under your feet would make the pose more challenging.

  (Note: If you don't have blocks, you can substitute them with large, thick hardcover books!)

- **Bolsters** - cushions that are often used for support and comfort in poses that require you to sit, kneel, or lie down on the ground.

  Bolsters can be rather pricey, but there are affordable options available as well.

  (Note: Alternatively, you can use throw pillows, blankets, or towels for cushioning.)

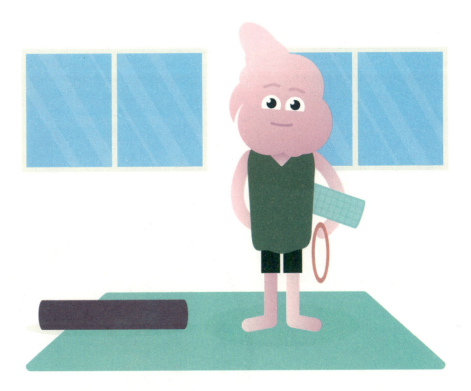

Choosing a Time & Place

The best way to integrate this new practice into your life and truly turn it into a habit is by thoughtfully designating a time and space for your practice.

It can also be helpful to **choose a trigger** — such as an alarm to remind you, a visual cue such as a sticky note, or anything else you find helpful — to accompany your yoga routine. Designating a trigger trains your brain to associate it with your yoga routine to help you stick to this new habit.

Ideally, the space you choose should be **quiet, comfortable, well-lit, and distraction-free.** Before each session, make sure the room temperature is comfortable and the area is clean and uncluttered.

The general rule of thumb is to have at least **20 square feet of open space to move around during your yoga session.** Having a mat can help you estimate how much space you need; mats are typically around 6 ft long and 2 ft wide, and you'll generally want to have another 1-2 ft of extra space around the entire mat.

Next, **figure out how your yoga practice will best fit your schedule**, which may take some experimentation. It's ideal to schedule your yoga session for the same time each day once you've found a time that works for you, but if your schedule tends to be irregular, it's okay to do it at different times so long as you're still consistently completing your sessions!

Yoga is equally beneficial at any time of the day, just try not to exercise too close to bedtime — too much movement and activity can stimulate your brain and make it harder to wind down.

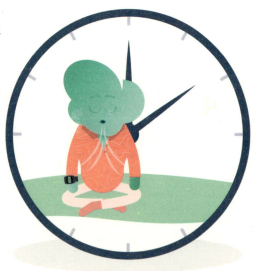

Before You Get Started...

You're almost ready to start your yoga practice! Before you go, here are a few super important points to keep in mind moving forward.

You've got this!

The Importance of Form & Alignment

Ensuring that you've got proper form and alignment is absolutely vital. Any time you're trying a new pose or movement, be sure you've read over how to complete them properly.

We'll provide step-by-step instructions for each pose/movement, as well as plenty of alignment cues. If you're ever feeling unclear, please take time to refer to those cues and instructions! Practicing yoga in front of a mirror is a great way to visualize your body and adjust your form as needed.

Without proper form and alignment:

- You risk **seriously** injuring yourself.
- You fail to engage and exercise the muscles that the pose/exercise is meant to target, which **greatly reduces the benefits** of the poses/exercises.
- Consistently **engaging and targeting the wrong muscles** through poor form eventually leads to muscle imbalances throughout the body.

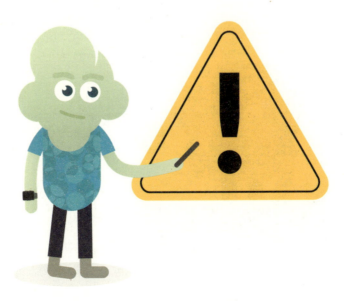

As with any other form of physical exercise, yoga carries a risk of injury without the proper precautions and considerations.

Before getting started, we recommend that you:

- **Consult your doctor** to make sure you're cleared to start, especially if you have any known medical conditions!

- Commit to **listening to your body and modifying poses** as needed! Do not push your body too far to get into a pose, especially if you start to experience any pain.

- Pay attention to your **nutrition, hydration, and overall wellness.** The exercise you get from your daily yoga flow is only one piece of the puzzle for achieving health and well-being. It won't help nearly as much if you're not taking good care of yourself the rest of the time!

Do's & Dont's

- **DO:** Hydrate before and after each yoga session (and throughout the day!)

- **DO:** Start with the basics, take your time, and work your way up to harder poses at a slow and steady pace.

- **DO:** If you're struggling, then modify, modify, modify! There's no shame whatsoever in modifying a pose to suit your experience or comfort levels.

- **DO:** Listen to your body and do what feels right for you!

- **DON'T:** Eat heavy meals before your yoga session.

- **DON'T:** Drink a lot of water during your workout. Stick with small sips instead!

- **DON'T:** Wear shoes or socks. Yoga is best practiced barefoot for stability and mobility in the ankles, feet, and toes.

- **DON'T:** Be absent-minded or distracted during your practice. Once your yoga session starts, challenge yourself to remain fully present and attentive throughout it.

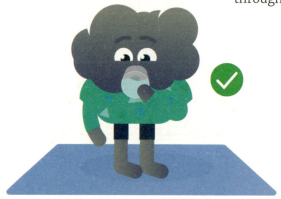

What To Expect

For the next 66 days, we'll provide you with a yoga routine for the day, as well as fresh daily content to help you stay engaged and committed to your goals, deepen your understanding of yoga, and expand your personal yoga practice.

This daily content comes in the form of pro-tips, in-depth exploration of various core concepts in yoga, food for thought, and resource recommendations — all of which will help you truly develop and master your personal yoga practice!

The daily content will also help you apply the core concepts you learn about, challenge you to overcome obstacles and try new things, and guide you to create a comprehensive personal yoga practice.

Daily Yoga Flows

We know everyone's time constraints, abilities, and goals are different, so each yoga routine contains three 15-minute segments — the Warm-Up, Peak Flow, & Cool Down. This allows you to choose whether your routine lasts 15, 30, or 45 minutes.

(**Note:** If you won't be doing the full routine, we recommend always having a warm-up of some sort, even if you shorten it a bit!)

We designed the yoga flows in this journey to start you at the basics and gradually increase in difficulty.

Take your time getting to know the poses, and feel free to repeat previous flows if you find that you're not quite ready to move on.

At the end of each flow, we've included an optional 5-minute meditative **Savasana**, which involves lying supine on the floor with your body completely relaxed and eyes closed. This is the perfect meditative way to end a yoga session, since it's so relaxing for the body and mind!

Your Action Plan for This Week

- [ ] **Read through the daily content** included with your routine each day to familiarize yourself with yoga and the process of developing a practice.

- [ ] **Commit wholeheartedly** to developing this habit by checking this journal daily and completing your yoga routines — no matter what!

- [ ] **Designate when and where you'll complete your yoga routine** each day. Experiment with different times to find what best suits your schedule if necessary.

- [ ] **Explore your capabilities and limitations** by being mindful and observant of how your body moves during your daily flow.

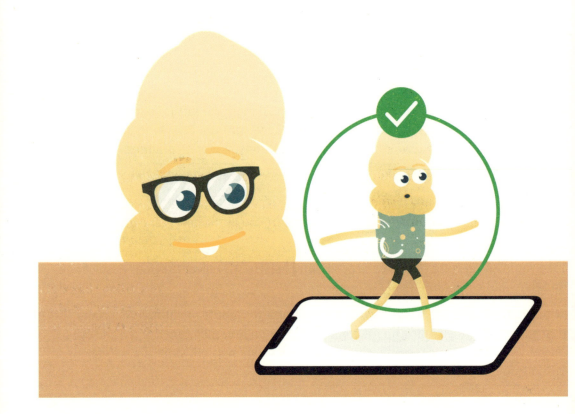

The Daily Content

Every single piece of content you're getting is a product of countless hours of sweat and research done by our team to ensure we're doing our best to:

1. Light a fire in you to succeed in adding the habit.
2. Provide you with the necessary knowledge and information to make developing your yoga practice simple and easy.
3. Make adding the habit fun and interesting.

Not only is every individual piece of content chosen amongst thousands of competing options, but as mentioned in the previous section, the order of the content has been creatively designed to get you through the struggles associated with the different stages of adding habits.

Here are the different types of content you can expect:

Pro-Tips

Pro-tips are the little golden nuggets of information you get to make implementing the habit on a day-to-day basis as simple and painless as possible. The point is to give you expert tips and hacks to get you going, and the variety and diversity of the different pro-tips will provide you with countless options for how to succeed in adding the habit.

Actionable Challenges

The Actionable Challenges you'll be receiving will be immensely important to your success in developing a consistent and substantive yoga practice.

Why?

They each target a different area of discipline that will help you force yourself to do what's right, especially when you don't feel like it.

By strengthening this willpower muscle inside you using small, very specific Actionable Challenges, your self-discipline will grow more and more every single day. These Actionable Challenges apply to all other aspects of your life — from curbing negative habits and distractions to building other healthy habits as well.

Favorite Resources

The useful resources you'll encounter include clips, podcasts, books, apps, websites, and anything else that we think will help make adding this habit to your day-to-day life much more seamless!

Connecting with people who have walked in your shoes and crossed over to the light will give you clear reference points that you can succeed at this, just as others, who have also struggled, have done. Watching, listening to, or reading inspirational and informational content will serve as the informative reminder you need to get started and push through your normal, expected struggles until you've mastered this

Food for Thought

Breaking the cycle of our own associative thinking is extremely difficult. It isn't easy to change the way we relate to any aspect of our lives - beginning a new yoga practice and adopting new perspectives is no different!

New ideas and perspectives are very helpful when it comes to changing the way we think and act. This content will provide you with an opportunity to evaluate how you think and shift perspectives if it seems useful.

Affirmations

Affirmations and visualization are highly effective tools used by some of the most successful people to have ever lived. From athletes to actors to CEOs, affirmations are used to help channel positive energy towards goals and create an inevitable connection between your present self and the end goal you have in mind.

What Affirmations Really Do

1. Subconsciously tap into your creativity muscle to begin generating creative ways of reaching your goals.

2. Subconsciously program your brain to associate yourself with the end goal you have in mind and prepare you to mentally sort out the steps necessary to get from where you are right now to your end goals.

3. Attract you to your goal by the simple act of envisioning yourself where you ultimately want to be.

4. Motivate you in the sense that it literally causes your brain to believe that you have within you the power, ability and capability to get exactly where you want in life.

So What Does It Mean to Use Affirmations?

Using affirmations is the act of repeating to yourself that you already are the person you want to be, envisioning that you can achieve your life goals, and you can be exactly the person you ideally hope to be.

It is the repeating of idealistic situations you would like to see yourself in, except you say them in the present tense, as if they were true now.

While repeating these affirmations, you visualize yourself as this ideal person, in the ideal situation you want to see yourself in, which trains your brain to believe it is possible.

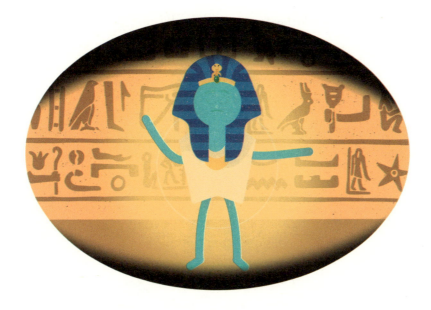

One Simple Idea

We hope that after reading the introductory pages, you're motivated and ready to tackle tomorrow with every ounce of energy you have.

We'll leave you to it with a breakdown of one simple idea...

1

Tomorrow, you will be exactly
who you are today.

2

The rest of your life is a future
projection of who you are today.

3

If you change today,
tomorrow will be different.

4

If you don't change today,
the rest of your life is predetermined.

Commit.

This week:
No matter what happens each day...

...whether I am exhausted
*or have the <u>**worst**</u> day of my life...*

...whether I win the lottery
*or have the <u>**best**</u> day of my life...*

*<u>I **will** stick to my yoga practice</u>*
for the next week.

*My word is like **gold**.*

I will do whatever it takes to make this happen.

I will stick to my yoga practice.

_____

Signature   Date

Phase 1: Flow 01 - 07

Hell Week

My main yoga goal for this phase:

Phase 1 Overview

When beginning a new habit, what's really important is getting to the point where you start to see the benefits you expect.

Starting won't be easy... You need to believe in yourself and take at least one concrete step in the direction of your goal every single day during this phase because it's really easy to lose hope right off the bat.

Make use of every tip, every affirmation, and all the motivation you're getting to make it as easy as possible to take just one action towards your goal every day.

Remember, we want to get to the point where we see benefits, and from that point on, self-motivation to re-acquire those benefits comes into play and smooths out the process.

Takeaways from this phase

❖ Designate a time and space for your yoga practice.

❖ Perform the daily yoga flows and start to develop a deep awareness of your body.

❖ Establish a clear purpose for developing your practice and set realistic goals.

❖ Begin cultivating an inner awareness of who you are and who you want to grow into through your practice.

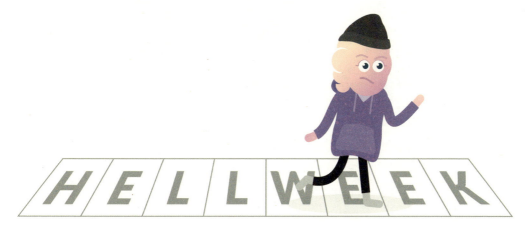

Pro-Tip

Asanas: learn & practice the poses individually.

If you're completely new to practicing yoga, or even if you just need a refresher, consider taking the time to look over and try out each pose individually.

Pay attention to how your body feels, your alignment, and the flow of your breath.

The more familiar these movements become to your body, the easier and smoother your daily yoga flow will be!

Every asana (pose) has four basic components:

- The Starting Position
- Entering the Pose
- Holding the Pose
- Releasing the Pose

Something as simple as being mindful and aware of these four components can deepen your practice, cultivate a mind-body connection, and help prevent injuries!

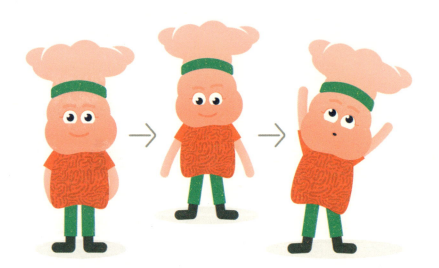

"Exercises are like prose, whereas yoga is the poetry of movements. Once you understand the grammar of yoga, you can write the poetry of your movements." - Amit Ray

Segment 1: Warm-Up

Full Session Exercise Guide:
habitnest.com/pages/yoga-day-1

1. Toe Flexion/Extension
30 sec.

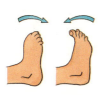

2. Ankle Rotations
30 sec.

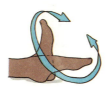

3. Seated Knee Rotations
30 sec. per side

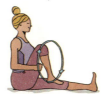

4. Cradle Pose
30 sec. per side

If you're rounding in the lower back, try placing a folded blanket or towel under your sit bones.

5. Seated Hip Rotations
30 sec. per side

Small circles with slow & controlled movement.

6. Seated Butterfly Wings
30-60 sec.

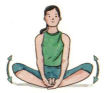

Gently pull the soles of the feet open.

7. Finger Abduction/Adduction
30 sec.

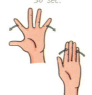

8. Wrist Flexion/Extension
30 sec.

9. Wrist Rotations
30 sec.

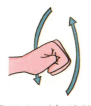

Rotate inward for 15-30 seconds, then outward.

10. Elbow Flexion/Extension
30 sec.

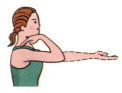

11. Shoulder Socket Rotations
30-60 sec.

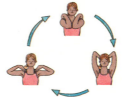

Slow and smooth movement!

12. Seated Neck Rolls
30 sec. each direction

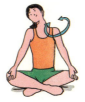

Sit up tall, release any tension in your shoulders, neck, or jaw, and take it slow.

13. Easy Pose Upward Salute
30-60 sec.

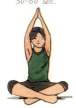

14. Easy Pose Side Bends
30 sec. per side

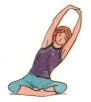

Keep your spine tall and your sit bones grounded.

15. Revolved Easy Pose
30 sec. per side

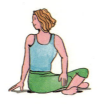

Keep your shoulders relaxed away from your neck and ears. Keep your chest broad.

16. Cat-Cow Pose
30-60 sec., alternating

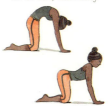

Knees align with hips. Hands align with shoulders. Thighs remain straight & tight.

Segment 2: Peak Flow

As you dive into the main portion of this first flow, consider carving out some extra time for this one - that way you can take it slow and familiarize yourself with the movements, instead of rushing it because of time constraints.

1. Mountain Pose
30-60 sec.

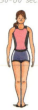

Keep muscles engaged w/o making your body stiff and rigid or locking any joints.

2. Chair Pose
30 sec.

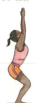

Try not to let your knees go past your toes; Neck and spine should be straight.

3. Standing Forward Fold
30-60 sec.

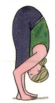

Bend at the hips. Spine should be long and straight.

4. Half Forward Fold Pose
15 sec.

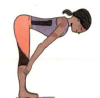

You can place your hands anywhere on the shins, but avoid placing your hands on the knees.

5. Plank Pose
30-60 sec.

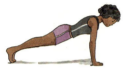

Keep a straight line from head to toe. Your core should be actively engaged.

6. Four-Limbed Staff Pose
30 sec.

See if you can lower yourself far enough that your shoulder blades are level with your elbows.

7. Upward-Facing Dog Pose
30 sec.

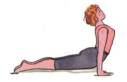

Avoid letting the shoulders creep up toward the ears.

8. Downward-Facing Dog
30-60 sec.

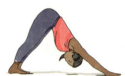

Aim to sink your heels as close to the ground as you can. Draw shoulders away from ears.

9. Warrior I Pose
30 sec. each side

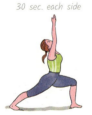

Keep core engaged by drawing your belly button inward toward the spine.

10. Plank Pose
30-60 sec.

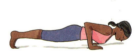

11. Four-Limbed Staff Pose
30 sec.

Remember, keep your elbows stacked above your wrists.

12. Upward-Facing Dog Pose
30-60 sec.

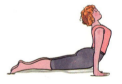

Don't let your shoulders shrug up toward your ears.

13. Downward-Facing Dog
30-60 sec.

Try to sink your heels a little lower with each exhale.

14. Half Forward Fold Pose
15 sec.

Remember, don't place your hands on or lock your knees!

15. Standing Forward Fold
30 sec.

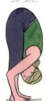

Take a slight bend in the knees and sway your upper body gently from side to side.

16. Chair Pose
30 sec.

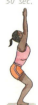

Keep thighs parallel to the floor for added challenge, but only if it feels right.

Segment 3: Cool Down

DATE

1. Easy Pose

30-60 sec.

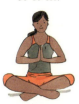

If this pose is uncomfortable for you, try placing a folded blanket underneath your sit bones!

2. Seated Cat-Cow

30-60 sec., alternating

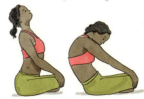

3. Revolved Easy Pose

30 sec. per side

Lengthen the tail bone toward the ground, creating a tall, straight spine. Chest stays broad.

4. Upward-Facing Seated Straddle

30-60 sec.

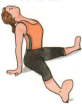

Knees pointing upward to the ceiling. Shoulder blades engaged to keep your chest open.

5. Seated Forward Fold Pose

60 sec.

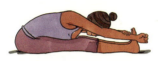

If you can't reach the sides of your feet, just grab on to your ankles or shins.

6. Wind Release Pose

60 sec.

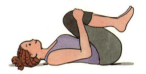

Keep the lower back grounded and shoulders firmly planted. Head and neck relaxed.

7. Happy Baby Pose

30-60 sec.

Make sure you're grabbing onto the outer sides of your feet, not the inner sides

8. Supine Spinal Twist II

30 sec. per side

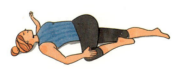

If you need to modify this pose, place a folded blanket/towel or a cushion under your knee.

9. Reclining Bound Angle Pose w/ Elbow Grab

30-60 sec.

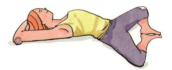

While in the pose, tuck your chin just enough to stretch and elongate the back of your neck.

10. Supine Butterfly Wings

30-60 sec.

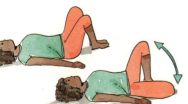

Keep your movements slow, controlled, and flowing smoothly with your breath.

11. Corpse Pose

5 mins

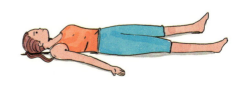

Pro-Tip

Asanas: create a strong foundation.

Many of the poses and flows you'll encounter require you to have a firm base of support, whether you're standing, sitting, or lying on your mat.

Balance and stability require plenty of core strength (which you'll build up along the way by completing your yoga flows), as well as good mobility in the hips and pelvis.

Your daily yoga flows will naturally increase your balance and stability, but it's also important to pay close attention to the way your hands and feet are positioned.

In standing poses, make sure your feet are firmly planted with your toes active and engaged. Keep all 4 corners of your feet grounded, and activate the muscles.

In poses that require your hands to bear weight, keep your palms flat, spread your fingers, and keep your arms strong, as if you were trying to push the floor away from you.

Your shoulders should remain back and down rather than shrugging up and in toward your ears.

Keep in mind that your joints should always be **stacked** (*i.e. shoulders stacked directly above wrists/hands, knees stacked above feet*) in order to engage the right muscles and prevent injury.

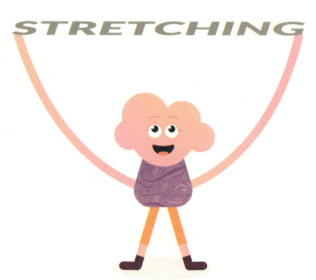

"Yoga practice can make us more and more sensitive to subtler and subtler sensations in the body. Paying attention to and staying with finer and finer sensations within the body is one of the surest ways to steady the wandering mind." - Ravi Ravindra

Segment 1: Warm-Up

Full Session Exercise Guide:
habitnest.com/pages/yoga-day-2

1. Constructive Rest Pose
30-60 sec.

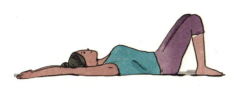

2. Cycling Pose
60-90 sec., alternating legs

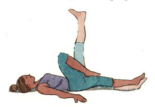

Avoid pulling your legs so close to your chest that it causes your back to flatten.

3. Supine Windshield Wipers
30 sec. per side

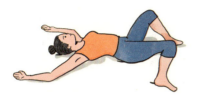

Keep your shoulder blades both firmly rooted to the ground throughout this exercise.

4. Reclined Half Cow Face Pose
30-60 sec. per side

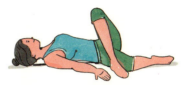

Keep your shoulder blades flat on the floor, and adjust this pose however you need to!

5. Reclined Hand-to-Big-Toe Pose
30 sec. per side

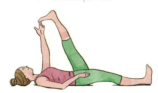

If you're struggling, bend the knee of the grounded leg and plant your foot flat on the floor.

6. Reverse Pigeon Pose
30 sec. per side

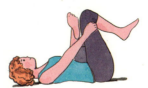

Be careful not to strain your knee! If you feel any pain or discomfort, relax the other leg back to the floor and very gently guide your knee out of the pose.

7. Supine Spinal Twist II Pose
30 sec. per side

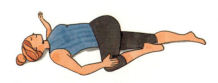

If you can't hook your foot behind the calf of the other leg, keep them crossed at the thighs.

8. Reclined Cow Face Pose
30 sec., then reverse legs & repeat

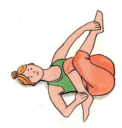

Shoulder blades stay flat on the floor, pulled away from each other. Keep back of hips flat.

Segment 2: Peak Flow

> Repeat poses 6-12, switching to the opposite side as necessary for asymmetrical poses.

1. Bound Angle Pose
60 sec.

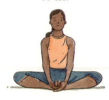

Gently pull the soles of the feet open as if you're opening a book. Helps the hips open!

2. Firelog Pose Variation
30 sec. per side

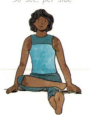

3. Half Cow Face Pose
30 sec. per side

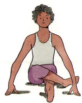

Remember to hinge from the hips and keep back long and straight.

4. Cow Face Pose w/ Eagle Arms
30 sec., then switch arms & legs

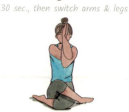

If you have difficulty with the Eagle Arms, place hands on the opposite shoulder (like a hug).

5. Mountain Pose
15 sec.

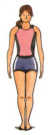

6. Mountain Pose w/ Beginner Eagle Arms
30 sec.

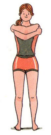

7. Warrior I Pose w/ Eagle Arms
30 sec.

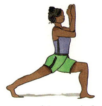

Keep your pelvis squarely facing forward and left thighbone pushed back away from you.

8. Chair Pose w/ Eagle Arms
30 sec.

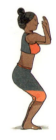

9. Eagle Pose
30 sec.

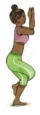

If this is difficult, keep legs together OR cross legs without hooking your foot behind your calf.

10. Chair Pose w/ Cactus Arms
30 sec.

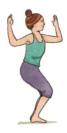

11. Warrior I Pose w/ Cactus Arms
30 sec.

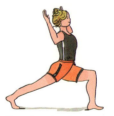

Keep chest broad and open, and shoulders down away from the ears.

12. Mountain Pose w/ Cactus Arms
30 sec.

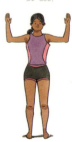

13. Garland Pose
30 sec.

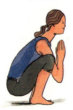

If you experience any knee strain in this pose, you can substitute this with a regular squat.

14. Wide Child's Pose
30-60 sec.

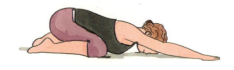

Keep your shoulder blades firmly in place, and make sure they don't shrug toward the ears.

Segment 3: Cool Down

DATE

1. Staff Pose
30-60 sec.

2. Half Lord of the Fishes Pose
30 sec. per side

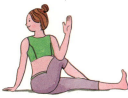

Remember to keep your chest broad and your shoulder blades strong!

3. Staff Pose w/ Feet Movements
30 sec.

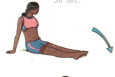

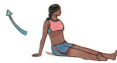

4. Fish Pose Backbend Flow
60 sec.

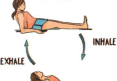
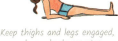

Keep thighs and legs engaged, and your heels pressing forward away from you.

5. Caterpillar Pose
30 sec.

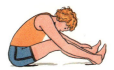

Keep the spine long & avoid rounding your back.

6. Seated Forward Fold Pose
30-60 sec.

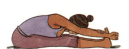
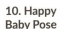
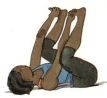

If you can't reach the sides of your feet, grab on to your ankles or shins.

7. Bridge Pose
30-60 sec.

Keep your feet hip-distance apart and grounded. Don't let your knees start drifting inward.

8. Half Wind Release Pose
30 sec. per side

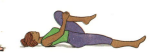

Only go as deep into this stretch as you feel comfortable with.

9. Wind Release Pose w/ Knee to Nose
30-60 sec.

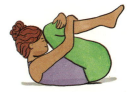

10. Happy Baby Pose
30-60 sec.

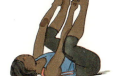

11. Full-Body Stretch Pose
30 sec.

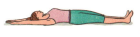

12. Banana Pose
30 sec. per side

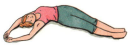

13. Supine Spinal Twist II Pose
30 sec. per side

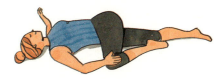

If you want a deeper spinal twist, rest one hand on your knee. Just let gravity do the work!

14. Corpse Pose
5 mins.

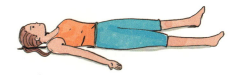

If you experience any head or neck discomfort, support your head with a folded blanket.

Food for Thought

Dharana: the importance of consistency & self-reflection.

As with any other habit, consistency is absolutely vital for establishing a yoga practice. Consistency is what allows us to build up the neural pathways required to truly make an action habitual (or, in other words, automatic).

That doesn't mean you have to consistently have a perfect yoga session by any means — what matters is that you consistently have a yoga session at all, even if it's shorter, simpler, or at a different time.

Make it a priority to develop this habit for your health and wellness.

As long as you're consistently doing something to stay on track, you'll have a successful practice!

Self-study and reflection will play a massive role in developing your yoga practice.

You will be challenged to look inward and get to know your true self, which involves learning to love, accept, and heal that true self hiding within you.

Bear in mind that this journey doesn't necessarily have to be spiritual for you.

Yoga isn't a religion, nor does it have to be about connecting to something divine; it's just a deeply personal journey to be experienced both on and off the mat through your practice and lifestyle.

YOU are the divine being you're trying to connect to!

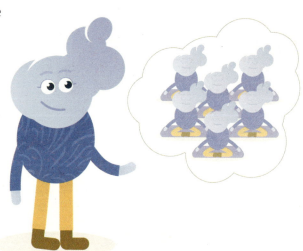

"The very heart of yoga practice is abhyasa - steady effort in the direction you want to go." - Sally Kempton

Segment 1: Warm-Up

Full Session Exercise Guide:
habitnest.com/pages/yoga-day-3

1. Easy Pose
30-60 sec.

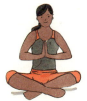

The underside of your chin should be parallel to the floor.

2. Seated Shoulder Rolls
30 sec. forward, then backward

3. Seated Neck Rolls
30 sec. each direction

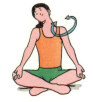

Be careful not to strain your neck. Keep your movements slow and controlled.

4. Seated Torso Circles
30 sec. each direction

5. Easy Pose Warm-Up
1-2 mins

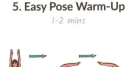
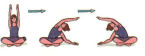

Remember to keep your sit bones grounded throughout this exercise. Take it slow if needed.

6. Cat-Cow Pose
30-60 sec., alternating

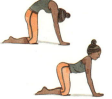

7. Table Top Hip Circles
30-45 sec. each direction

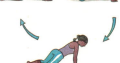

8. Kneeling Sun Salutation
1-2 mins

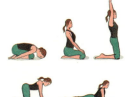

9. Staff Pose
30 sec.

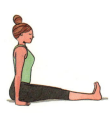

10. Revolved Staff Pose Flow
30-60 sec., alternating

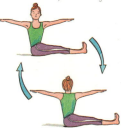

11. Staff Pose Leg Lift & Slide
30 sec. per side

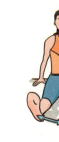

12. Staff Pose Knee Stretch
30 sec. per side

13. Seated Hip Rotations
30 sec. per side

14. Cradle Pose
30 sec. per side

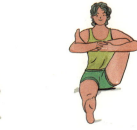

If you experience rounding in the low back, place a folded towel under your sit bones.

15. Seated Straddle Pose
30-60 sec.

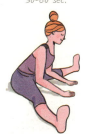

Keep an eye on your leg positioning - your knees should be pointing upward to the ceiling.

16. Head-to-Knee Pose
30 sec. per side

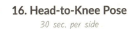
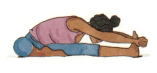

Segment 2: Peak Flow

> Repeat poses 1-8, switching to the opposite side as necessary for asymmetrical poses.

1. Downward-Facing Dog Pose
30 sec.

2. Low Lunge Pose
30 sec.

3. High Lunge Pose
30 sec.

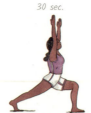

4. Warrior II Pose
30 sec.

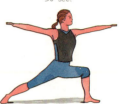

Sink your heels a little lower with each exhale.

Keep your pelvis square and try not to move your knee forward past your toes.

Don't let your left thigh bone drop! Keep it pressed back with your pelvis squarely forward.

Keep stance wide enough that your wrists approximately line up with your ankles.

5. Humble Warrior Pose
30 sec.

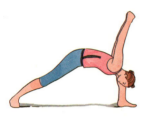

6. Goddess Pose
30-45 sec.

7. Five-Pointed Star Pose
30 sec.

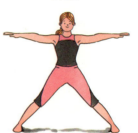

8. Vinyasa I
30-45 sec.

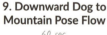

Make sure you tuck your tailbone forward, knit the bottom ribs in, and engage your core.

9. Downward Dog to Mountain Pose Flow
60 sec.

10. Volcano Pose Namaste Salute
30 sec.

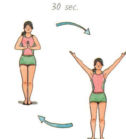

11. Upward Salute to Forward Fold Flow
30-60 sec.

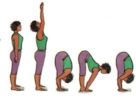

12. Plank Pose
30 sec.

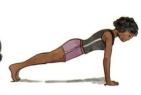

13. Locust Pose
30-60 sec.

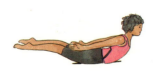

14. Thunderbolt Pose
30-60 sec.

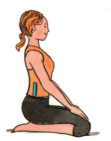

15. Kneeling Pose
30 sec.

16. Camel Pose
30 sec.

Lift your upper body with your sternum, not your chin. Back of the neck should stay long.

If you're struggling with this pose, stay in Kneeling Pose and try to deepen the backbend.

Segment 3: Cool Down

DATE

1. Wide Child's Pose
30-60 sec.

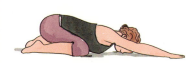

2. Camel Pose w/ Hands to Floor
30 sec.

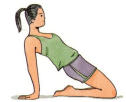

Keep your tailbone tucked slightly forward and your core engaged.

3. Camel Pose
30 sec.

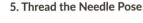

4. Puppy Dog Pose
30-60 sec.

5. Thread the Needle Pose
30 sec. per side

6. Table Top to Child's Pose
30-60 sec.

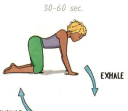

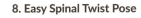
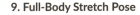

7. Staff Pose
30-60 sec.

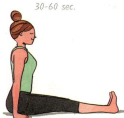

8. Easy Spinal Twist Pose
30 sec. per side

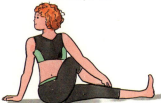

9. Full-Body Stretch Pose
30 sec.

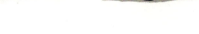

10. Supine Spinal Twist II Pose
30 sec. per side

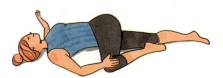

11. Corpse Pose
5 mins

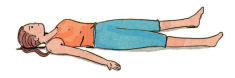

Psssstt... We like rewarding people (like you) who TAKE ACTION and actually use this journal. Email us now at secret+yoga@habitnest.com for a secret gift ;)

Pro-Tip

Dhyana: entering & maintaining a meditative state.

If you're new to meditation, you may find it easier to incorporate it into your yoga practice if you spend some time acclimating to it outside of your daily flows.

There are no hard-and-fast rules regarding when, where, or how to meditate, but **try setting aside time this week to practice meditation** (even just 5-10 minutes a day!).

Choose somewhere comfortable, quiet, and private where you can sit or lie down.

One of the hardest things for the mind to do is absolutely nothing. We're wired to be thought-machines and we live in a world of constant stimulation, so of course, we can't expect our stream of thoughts to completely shut off without practice!

One thing to keep in mind that you might find helpful.

- **Don't fight or resist the thoughts/feelings that arise.** The more frustrated you get that your mind isn't clear, the more difficult it becomes to reach/maintain a meditative state. It's also not uncommon for beginners to experience some anxiety or irritability at first.

Simply acknowledge the thoughts/feelings, allow them a moment to pass, then allow them to float away.

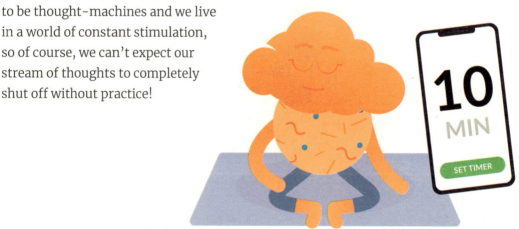

"True meditation is about being fully present with everything that is, including discomfort and challenges. It is not an escape from life." - Craig Hamilton

Segment 1: Warm-Up

Full Session Exercise Guide:
habitnest.com/pages/yoga-day-4

1. Thunderbolt Pose w/ Torso Twists
30-60 sec.

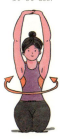

2. Thunderbolt Pose w/ Swinging Arms
30-60 sec.

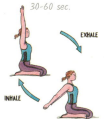

Make sure you keep your shoulder blades down away from your ears.

3. Thunderbolt Pose w/ Eagle Arms
30 sec., switch arms & repeat

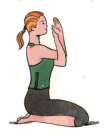

4. Cat-Cow Pose
30-60 sec., alternating

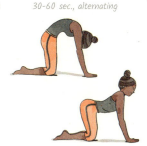

5. Sphinx Pose
30-60 sec.

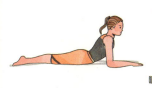

6. Rowing the Boat
30-60 sec.

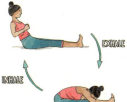

7. Fish Pose Backbend Flow
60 sec.

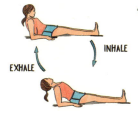

8. Boat Pose Roll-Ups
30-60 sec.

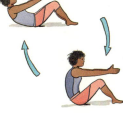

9. Full-Body Stretch to Seated Forward Fold Flow
30-60 sec.

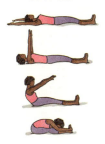

10. Cow Face Pose
30 sec., then switch arms & legs

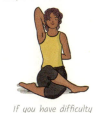

If you have difficulty achieving the Cow Face arms, grab onto a towel or strap.

11. Seated Neck Rolls
30 sec. each direction

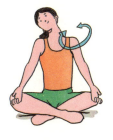

12. Seated Shoulder Rolls
30 sec. forward, then backward

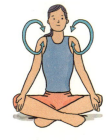

13. Seated Torso Circles
30 sec. each direction

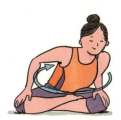

14. Seated Deltoid Stretch
30 sec. per side

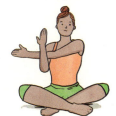

15. Cradle Pose
30 sec. per side

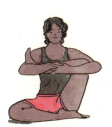

16. Easy Pose Side Bend
30 sec. per side

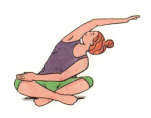

Be sure to keep your sit bones grounded the whole time!

Segment 2: Peak Flow

> Repeat poses 6-12, switching to the opposite side as necessary for asymmetrical poses.

1. Bound Angle Pose
60 sec.
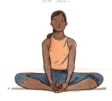

2. Firelog Pose
30 sec. per side
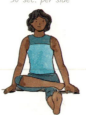

3. Half Cow Face Pose
30 sec. per side
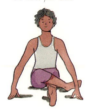

4. Cow Face Pose w/ Eagle Arms
30 sec., then switch arms & legs
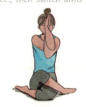

5. Mountain Pose
15 sec.
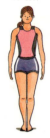

6. Mountain Pose w/ Beginner Eagle Arms
30 sec.
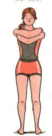

7. Warrior I Pose w/ Eagle Arms
30 sec.
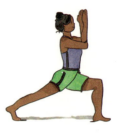

8. Chair Pose w/ Eagle Arms
30 sec.

9. Eagle Pose
30 sec.

10. Chair Pose w/ Cactus Arms
30 sec.
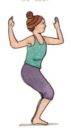

11. Warrior I Pose w/ Cactus Arms
30 sec.
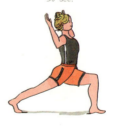

12. Mountain Pose w/ Cactus Arms
30 sec.
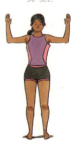

13. Garland Pose
30 sec.
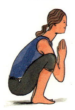

14. Wide Child's Pose
30-60 sec.
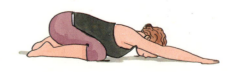

Segment 3: Cool Down

DATE

1. Toe Squat
30-60 sec.

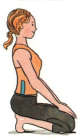

2. Toe Squat w/ Head-to-Knees
30 sec.

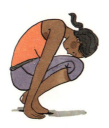

3. Standing Forward Fold
30 sec.

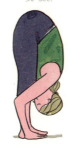

4. Standing Roll-Up Flow
30-60 sec.

5. Volcano Pose
30-60 sec.

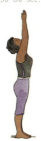

6. Swaying Palm Tree Pose
30 sec. per side

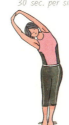

Even as you lean, keep your legs and pelvis strong and aligned.

7. Standing Bound Locust Pose
30-60 sec.

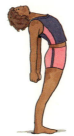

8. Dangling Pose
30-60 sec.

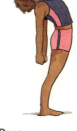

9. Revolved Forward Fold w/ Bent Knee
30 sec. per side

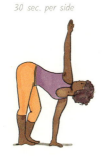

10. Garland Pose
30 sec.

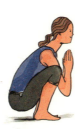

11. Seated Wind Release Pose
30-60 sec.

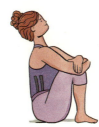

12. Spinal Rock Pose
30-60 sec.

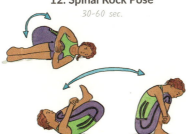

If you feel discomfort, come onto your back and bring your head to your knees.

13. Corpse Pose
5 mins.

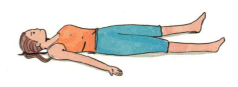

Pro-Tip

Pratyahara: Tips for turning your space into a yoga sanctuary.

Part of Pratyahara involves creating the right environment for your practice, so it's great to have a space that helps you feel both comfortable and focused. Your yoga space should make you feel completely at-ease and free your mind from distractions.

The biggest factor to consider is how much space you have. It's recommended to have at least 20 square feet of space, but as long as you can comfortably perform the poses without hitting nearby objects, any space will do.

For modern Yogis, devices of any sort can be extremely distracting. Put your phone on silent and leave it somewhere out of sight, turn digital clocks to face away from you, and turn off any other nearby devices (TVs, computers/laptops, etc.).

When it comes to decorating your yoga space, simplicity is the way to go. Keep the space clean and clutter-free, and avoid harsh lighting.

Adding a large mirror can help the room feel more open and bright, as well as allow you to check your alignment during flows.

If you're looking to change up the decor, try adding:

- A **wicker basket** to store your mat and/or small props (towels, blocks, strap, bolster, etc.)
- An **indoor plant** (bonus points for plants that help to purify the air, like bamboo palm or gerbera daisies)
- A **small shelf or table** to hold your speaker, water bottle, or other small items.

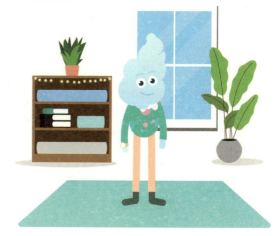

"Yoga is not a work-out, it's a work-in, and this is the point of spiritual practice; to make us teachable, to open up our hearts and focus our awareness so that we can know what we already know and be who we already are." - Rolf Gates

Segment 1: Warm-Up

Full Session Exercise Guide:
habitnest.com/pages/yoga-day-5

1. Corpse Pose
60 sec.

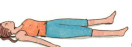

2. Banana Pose
30 sec. per side

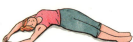

3. Wind Release Pose
60 sec.

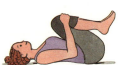

4. Circle of Joy
60 sec.

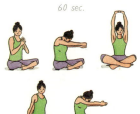

5. Cat-Cow Pose
30-60 sec., alternating

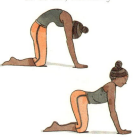

6. Tiger Pose
30 sec. per side

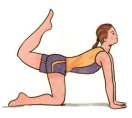

7. Child's Pose w/ Arms to One Side
30 sec. per side

Keep your shoulder blades firmly in place, and make sure they don't shrug toward the ears.

8. Child's Pose Sun Salutation
1-2 mins.

9. Thunderbolt Pose w/ Swinging Arms
30-60 sec.

10. Shoulder Socket Rotations
30-60 sec.

11. Cow Face Arms
30 sec., switch arms & repeat

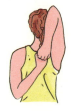

If you have difficulty achieving the Cow Face arms, grab onto a towel or strap.

12. Standing Forward Fold Pose
30 sec.

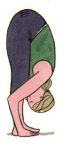

13. Standing Roll-Up Flow
30-60 sec.

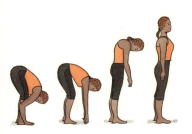

14. Standing Circle of Joy
60 sec.

15. Breath of Joy
30-60 sec.

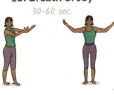

Segment 2: Peak Flow

> Repeat poses 1-8, switching to the opposite side as necessary for asymmetrical poses.

1. Downward-Facing Dog Pose
30 sec.

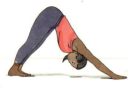

Try to sink your heels a little lower with each exhale.

2. Low Lunge Pose
30 sec.

3. High Lunge Pose
30 sec.

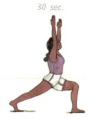

4. Warrior II Pose
30 sec.

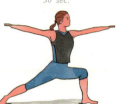

5. Humble Warrior Pose
30 sec.

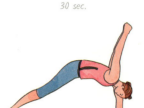

6. Goddess Pose
30-45 sec.

Make sure you tuck your tailbone forward, knit the bottom ribs in, and engage your core.

7. Five-Pointed Star Pose
30 sec.

8. Vinyasa I
30-45 sec.

9. Downward Dog to Mountain Pose Flow
60 sec.

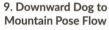

10. Volcano Pose Namaste Salute
30 sec.

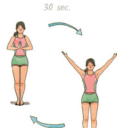

11. Upward Salute to Forward Fold Flow
30-60 sec.

12. Plank Pose
30 sec.

13. Locust Pose
30-60 sec.

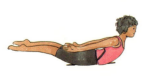

Lift your upper body with your sternum, not your chin. Back of the neck should stay long.

14. Thunderbolt Pose
30-60 sec.

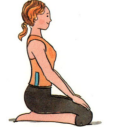

15. Kneeling Pose
30 sec.

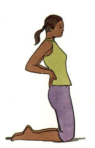

16. Camel Pose
30 sec.

Segment 3: Cool Down

DATE

1. Child's Pose

30-60 sec.

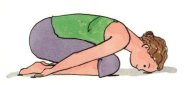

2. Half Lord of the Fishes Pose

30 sec. per side

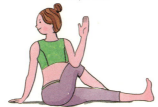

Remember to keep your chest broad and your shoulder blades strong!

3. Staff Pose w/ Feet Movements

30 sec.

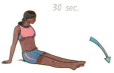

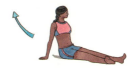

4. Staff Pose w/ Hands Back

15-30 sec.

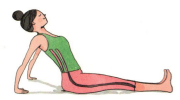

5. Upward Plank Pose

30-60 sec.

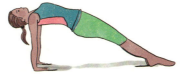

6. Seated Forward Fold Pose

60 sec.

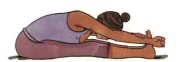

7. Wind Release Pose

60 sec.

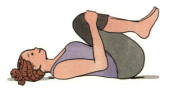

8. Bridge Pose

30-60 sec.

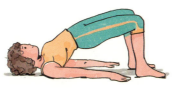

9. Supine Spinal Twist II Pose

30 sec. per side

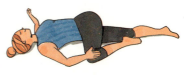

10. Happy Baby Pose

30-60 sec.

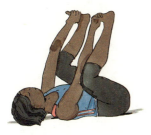

11. Reclining Bound Angle Pose w/ Elbow Grab

30-60 sec.

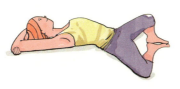

Tuck your chin just enough to stretch and elongate the back of your neck.

12. Corpse Pose

5 mins.

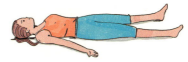

Pro-Tip

Asanas: savor the Savasana.

No yoga session is quite complete without a Savasana (pronounced Shavasana)! As you may have noticed, each daily yoga routine includes an optional 5-minute Savasana; lying supine on your mat in Corpse Pose and focusing your attention on progressively relaxing every muscle in the body one by one.

This gives your body and mind a chance to relax, recover, and regroup, allowing you to face the rest of the day feeling both energized and calm. Evidence suggests that Savasana is helpful for decreasing stress, depression, insomnia, headaches, and blood pressure levels.

It's not uncommon to run into some resistance from your body and mind. You may have more muscle tension than you thought, struggle to fully relax some areas, or have a relaxed body but an overactive mind.

If you're having trouble getting fully relaxed and comfortable, try using folded blankets, towels, or cushions.

<u>Try to pinpoint which areas you're having trouble with and adjust your cushioning/support accordingly:</u>

- Place it under your head and neck for support. Your forehead should be slightly higher than your chin.

- Place it under your knees to reduce tension in the lower back.

- Place an eye mask or soft cloth over your eyes to help relax them and block out bright lights.

- To help relax your core, place a pillow or a couple of folded blankets/towels horizontally across your abdomen.

Seriously, take advantage of this built-in meditative practice whenever possible!

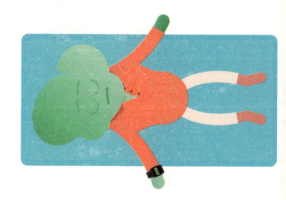

"Yoga is a dance between control and surrender — between pushing and letting go — and when to push and when to let go becomes part of the creative process, part of the open-ended exploration of your being." - Joel Kramer

Segment 1: Warm-Up

Full Session Exercise Guide:
habitnest.com/pages/yoga-day-6

1. Thunderbolt Pose w/ Torso Twists
30-60 sec.

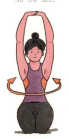

2. Thunderbolt Pose w/ Swinging Arms
30-60 sec.

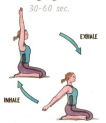

Make sure you keep your shoulder blades down away from your ears.

3. Thunderbolt Pose w/ Eagle Arms
30 sec., switch arms & repeat

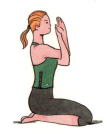

4. Cat-Cow Pose
30-60 sec., alternating

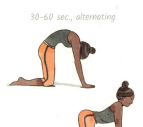

5. Sphinx Pose
30-60 sec.

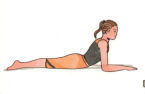

6. Rowing the Boat
30-60 sec.

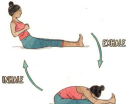

7. Fish Pose Backbend Flow
60 sec.

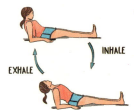

8. Boat Pose Roll-Ups
30-60 sec.

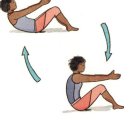

9. Full-Body Stretch to Seated Forward Fold Flow
30-60 sec.

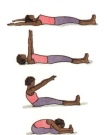

10. Cow Face Pose
30 sec., then switch arms & legs

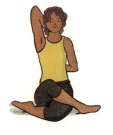

11. Seated Neck Rolls
30 sec. each direction

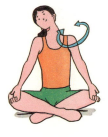

12. Seated Shoulder Rolls
30 sec. forward, then backward

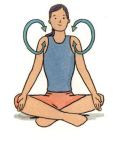

13. Seated Torso Circles
30 sec. each direction

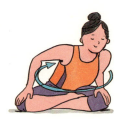

14. Seated Deltoid Stretch
30 sec. per side

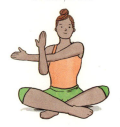

15. Cradle Pose
30 sec. per side

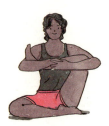

16. Easy Pose Side Bend
30 sec. per side

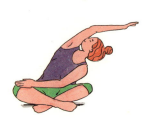

Segment 2: Peak Flow

1. Revolved Figure Four Pose
30-60 sec. per side

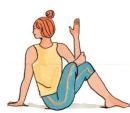

2. Sitting Swan Pose
30 sec. per side

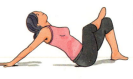

Be sure to lean back at the hips instead of the waist to avoid rounding your back.

3. Reverse Table Top Pose
30 sec.

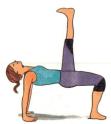

Keep your core engaged. Don't let your pelvis start to creep back down to the floor!

4. One-Legged Reverse Table Top Pose
30 sec. per side

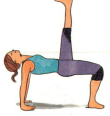

5. Upward Plank Pose
30-60 sec.

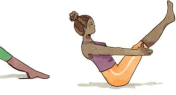

6. Boat Pose
30-60 sec.

It's crucial to make sure that you're still breathing even though your core is working hard!

7. Reclined Eagle Crunches
30-60 sec.

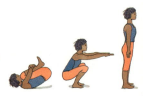

8. Wind Release to Mountain Pose Flow
30-60 sec.

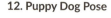

9. Chair Pose
30 sec.

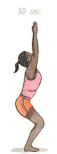

10. Standing Forward Fold Pose
30 sec.

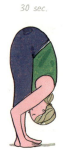

11. Plank to Downward Dog Pose Flow
30 sec.

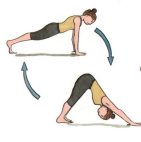

12. Puppy Dog Pose
30-60 sec.

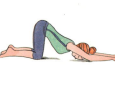

13. Revolved Downward-Facing Dog Pose
30 sec. per side

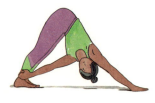

14. Garland Pose
30 sec.

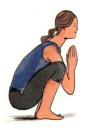

15. Revolved Squat Pose
30 sec. per side

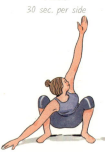

16. Wide Child's Pose
30-60 sec.

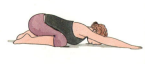

Segment 3: Cool Down

DATE

1. Child's Pose w/ Reverse Prayer
30-60 sec.

2. Table Top Pose
30 sec.

If this pose hurts your wrists or knees, place a folded blanket underneath them for padding.

3. Thread the Needle Pose
30 sec. per side

Keep your chest broad throughout this pose. Your movements should be slow and controlled.

4. Staff Pose
60 sec.

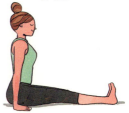

5. Sage Marichi Pose C
30 sec. per side

6. Seated Forward Fold
60 sec.

7. Bound Angle Pose
60 sec.

8. Seated Star Pose
60 sec.

9. Wind Release Pose
60 sec.

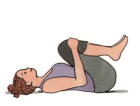

10. Half Plow Pose
30-60 sec.

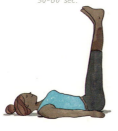

11. Bridge Pose
30-60 sec.

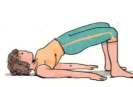

12. Supine Spinal Twist II Pose
30 sec. per side

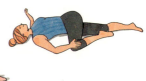

13. Reclining Bound Angle Pose
30-60 sec.

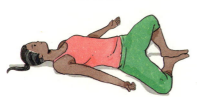

14. Corpse Pose
5 mins.

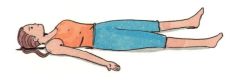

Feel free to experiment; you can situate your heels farther from or closer to your groin.

Actionable Challenge

Pranayama: intro to Pranayama & breathwork.

Breathwork is equally as important as the asanas for developing your yoga practice, as well as being valuable off the mat. It nourishes your body, soothes your mind, and brings your awareness back to the present.

Pranayama is the limb of yoga that focuses on harnessing and controlling your breath through exercises and techniques.

In Yogic tradition, your prana is said to be your life force. Pranayama aims to supercharge that life force and clear away any blockages so that your mind and body can achieve peak performance!

Throughout this journey, we'll introduce you to several popular Pranayama exercises to add to your tool belt and practice during your daily flow.

Let's start with the most basic technique: breathing with your diaphragm!

With this method, your diaphragm contracts downward to create more space in the chest cavity for your lungs to fill up and expand.

Give it a shot!

1. Sit or lie down somewhere comfortable. Keep your spine straight and long.
2. Place one hand on your chest near your heart, and place the other hand on your belly near the navel.
3. Slowly inhale through your nose, allowing your belly to expand rather than your chest.
4. Slightly part your lips and exhale slowly, allowing your belly and hand to sink back down.
5. Practice this breathing method for 2-3 minutes (or more!).

Actionable Challenge Completed: ☐

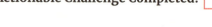

"When the breath control is correct, mind control is possible." - Pattabhi Jois

Segment 1: Warm-Up

Full Session Exercise Guide:
habitnest.com/pages/yoga-day-7

1. Easy Pose
30-60 sec.

2. Easy Pose Warm-Up
1-2 mins.

3. Cat-Cow to Child's Pose Flow
1-2 mins.

4. Thread the Needle Flow
30 sec. per side

5. Table Top Pose w/ Leg Raise
30 sec. per side

6. Supported Side Plank
30 sec. per side

7. Low Lunge w/ Hands to Knee
30 sec. per side

8. Easy Half Bow Pose
30 sec. per side

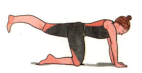
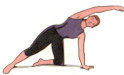
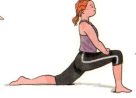
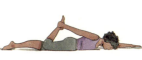

If there's hip discomfort, shift weight onto the back leg.

9. Vinyasa I
30-45 sec.

10. Mountain Pose
30 sec.

11. Standing Wind Release Pose
30 sec. per side

12. Mountain Pose w/ Twist
30 sec. per side

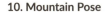
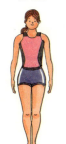
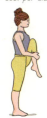
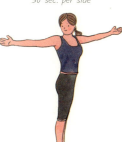

For added balance, feel free to use a wall, desk, chair, or other support option available.

13. Standing Backbend Pose
30-60 sec.

14. Standing Forward Fold w/ Knees Bent
30-60 sec.

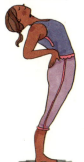
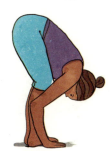

Segment 2: Peak Flow

1. Revolved Figure Four Pose
30-60 sec. per side

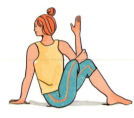

2. Sitting Swan Pose
30 sec. per side

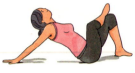

3. Reverse Table Top Pose
30 sec.

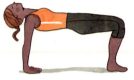

4. One-Legged Reverse Table Top Pose
30 sec. per side

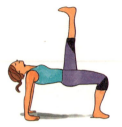

5. Upward Plank Pose
30-60 sec.

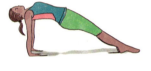

6. Boat Pose
30-60 sec.

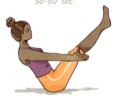

7. Reclined Eagle Crunches
30-60 sec.

8. Wind Release to Mountain Pose Flow
30-60 sec.

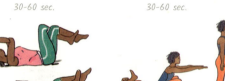

9. Chair Pose
30 sec.

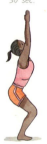

10. Standing Forward Fold Pose
30 sec.

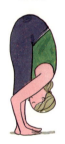

11. Plank to Downward Dog Pose Flow
30 sec.

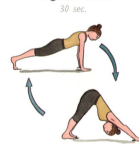

12. Puppy Dog Pose
30-60 sec.

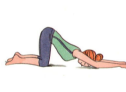

13. Revolved Downward-Facing Dog Pose
30 sec. per side

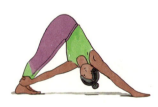

14. Garland Pose
30 sec.

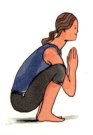

15. Revolved Squat Pose
30 sec. per side

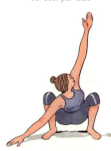

16. Wide Child's Pose
30-60 sec.

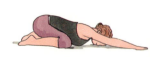

Segment 3: Cool Down

DATE

1. Toe Squat
30-60 sec.

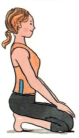

2. Toe Squat w/ Head-to-Knees
30 sec.

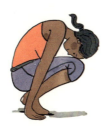

3. Standing Forward Fold
30 sec.

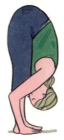

4. Standing Roll-Up Flow
30-60 sec.

5. Volcano Pose
30-60 sec.

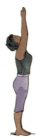

6. Swaying Palm Tree Pose
30 sec. per side

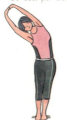

Even as you lean, keep your legs and pelvis strong and aligned.

7. Standing Bound Locust Pose
30-60 sec.

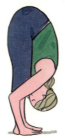

8. Dangling Pose
30-60 sec.

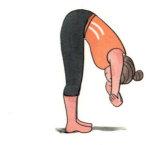

9. Revolved Forward Fold w/ Bent Knee
30 sec. per side

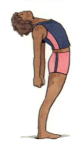

10. Garland Pose
30 sec.

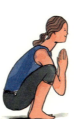

11. Seated Wind Release Pose
30-60 sec.

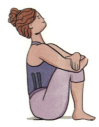

12. Spinal Rock Pose
30-60 sec.

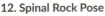
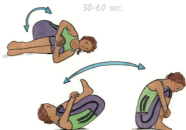

If you feel discomfort, come onto your back and bring your head to your knees.

13. Corpse Pose
5 mins.

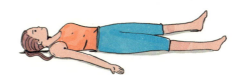

Recap Questions

1. Which parts of my body have had the most tightness, tension, or discomfort? Which parts of my body seemed to move smoothly or effortlessly?

2. Which poses seemed to feel more beneficial or alleviated the most pain/discomfort? How did that impact how I felt (mentally or physical) beyond the mat in everyday life?

3. Are there any noticeable muscle imbalances (i.e. one side is stronger or more flexible) between the muscles on my right compared to my left? Which muscles need to be tightened or stretched?

4. Do any of my daily habits contribute to muscle imbalances, tension, or strain? What can I do to be more mindful of those habits and shift toward positive ones?

5. What mental, emotional, or spiritual changes have I encountered thus far in my yoga practice? How have these changes impacted the rest of my life?

Phase 1 Done.

Phase 2: Flow 08 - 21

Digging Deep & Staying Consistent

My main yoga goal for this phase:

Phase 2 Overview

You've finished Hell Week and established a solid foundation to build your practice! Give yourself a gentle hug and take a moment to celebrate your progress. You deserve it!

Many of the principles in yoga challenge you to dig deep down to the core of who you are, reflect on what you find, and identify areas for growth and improvement.

It will likely be uncomfortable or a bit difficult at first, but as long as you stay committed and consistent, the reward you'll gain is absolutely priceless!

Show up to the mat and log it here in the journal every day, even for a short or imperfect session, no matter what. Consistency is more important than ever in this phase, so schedule and prioritize these precious moments on the mat.

This is YOUR time to love, understand, and nurture your mind and body, so show up for yourself!

Let's get growing!

Takeaways from this phase

❖ Turn your attention inward to understand yourself and eliminate distractions.

❖ Develop your ability to enter a deep meditative state.

❖ Work on controlling your breath & synchronizing it with your movements.

❖ Learn more about the core principles of yoga.

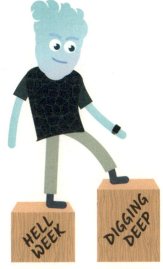
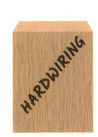

Food for Thought

Yamas: Ahimsa (non-violence).

Ahimsa is a foundational ethical principle of yoga that translates to "absence of injury."

It's all about doing no harm to ourselves, others, and our environment.

At face value, it seems like a piece of cake principle to follow — but it's much easier said than done.

For starters, this isn't just about causing physical harm, but also mental/emotional harm. It involves doing away with all of our habits, actions, or behaviors that bring harm in any form.

According to a set of ancient texts called the Vedas, harm comes in 3 main forms:

- **Kayaka** — Translates to "of the hand", meaning physical actions.
- **Vācaka** — Translates to "expressive", meaning through words, tones, and behaviors.
- **Manasika** — Translates to "of the mind", meaning harmful thoughts.

Aside from trying to limit your harmful actions, the best way to practice Ahimsa is to be the light that the world needs; show everyone you come across genuine kindness, compassion, and empathy.

It's also important to show **yourself** love and kindness. The way we think and speak about ourselves matters immensely, and Ahimsa requires that we do away with that negative self-talk.

Do no harm to yourself; make time for self-care, take it easy on yourself, and work on changing the negative inner voice into a positive one.

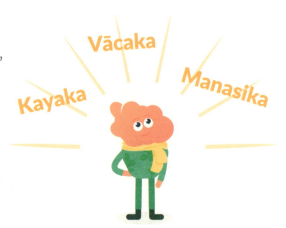

"Undisturbed calmness of mind is attained by cultivating friendliness toward the happy, compassion for the unhappy, delight in the virtuous, and indifference toward the wicked." - Patañjali

Segment 1: Warm-Up

Full Session Exercise Guide:
habitnest.com/pages/yoga-day-8

1. Toe Flexion/ Extension
30 sec.
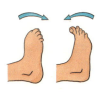

2. Ankle Rotations
30 sec.
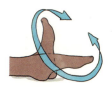

3. Seated Knee Rotations
30 sec. per side
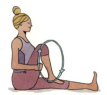

4. Cradle Pose
30 sec. per side
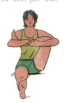

5. Seated Hip Rotations
30 sec. per side
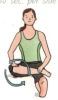

6. Seated Butterfly Wings
30-60 sec.
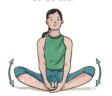

7. Finger Abduction/ Adduction
30 sec.

8. Wrist Flexion/ Extension
30 sec.
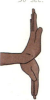

9. Wrist Rotations
30 sec.
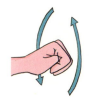

10. Elbow Flexion/ Extension
30 sec.
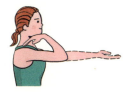

11. Shoulder Socket Rotations
30-60 sec.
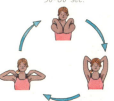

12. Seated Neck Rolls
30 sec. each direction
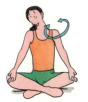

13. Easy Pose Upward Salute
30-60 sec.
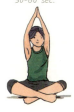

14. Easy Pose Side Bends w/ Fingers Interlocked
30 sec. per side

15. Revolved Easy Pose
30 sec. per side

16. Cat-Cow Pose
30-60 sec., alternating
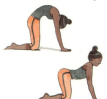

Segment 2: Peak Flow

> Repeat poses 1-4, switching to the opposite side as necessary for asymmetrical poses.

1. Plank to Downward Dog Pose Flow
30 sec.

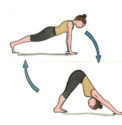

2. Three-Legged Downward Dog to Tiger Curl Flow
30 sec.

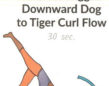

3. Lizard Pose
30-60 sec.

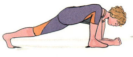

Keep your core engaged and your tailbone tucked forward slightly.

4. Sleeping Swan Pose
30-60 sec.

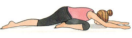

If you're not ready for this pose yet, try curling your back toes to lift the back leg.

5. Plank to Downward Dog Pose Flow
30 sec.

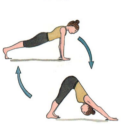

6. Standing Forward Fold Pose
30 sec.

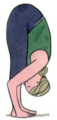

7. Extended Mountain Pose Backbend
30 sec.

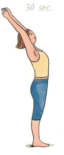

8. Mountain Pose Backbend w/ Cactus Arms
30 sec.

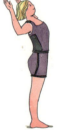

9. Garland Pose w/ Hands Forward
30 sec.

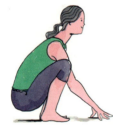

10. Staff Pose
30 sec.

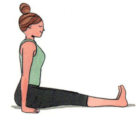

11. Bridge Pose w/ Arm Flow
30-60 sec.

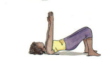

12. Half Plow Pose Flow
30-60 sec.

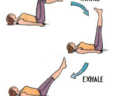

If needed, place a folded blanket/towel underneath your hips/lower back for support.

13. Shoulderstand Pose
30-60 sec.

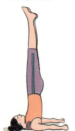

Do not try unless you absolutely feel ready and comfortable that you can even attempt this without hurting yourself.

14. Wind Release Pose
60 sec.

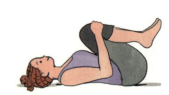

Segment 3: Cool Down

DATE

1. Staff Pose
30-60 sec.

2. Half Lord of the Fishes Pose
30 sec. per side

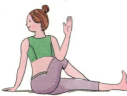

Remember to keep your chest broad and your shoulder blades strong!

3. Staff Pose w/ Feet Movements
30 sec.

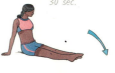

4. Fish Pose Backbend Flow
60 sec.

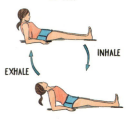

5. Caterpillar Pose
30 sec.

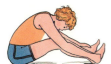

6. Seated Forward Fold Pose
30-60 sec.

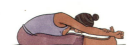

7. Bridge Pose
30-60 sec.

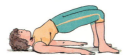

8. Half Wind Release Pose
30 sec. per side

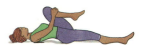

9. Wind Release Pose w/ Knee to Nose
30-60 sec.

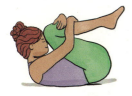

10. Happy Baby Pose
30-60 sec.

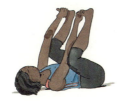

11. Full-Body Stretch Pose
30 sec.

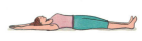

12. Banana Pose
30 sec. per side

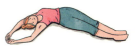

13. Supine Spinal Twist II Pose
30 sec. per side

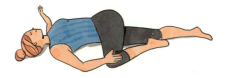

14. Corpse Pose
5 mins.

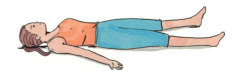

Food for Thought

Niyamas: Saucha (cleanliness/purity).

This Niyama focuses on cleanliness and purity in all aspects of life; your body, your diet, your thoughts, your words, your behavior, and even your environment.

Purity, in this case, doesn't mean holy or spiritual — it simply means free of bad/harmful things!

You can practice Saucha in many ways, including:

- Keeping up with your hygiene
- Wearing clean clothes
- Keeping your environment clean and free of clutter
- Eating clean, healthy foods
- Try replacing negative thoughts with positive ones
- Speak kindly to yourself and others

A common saying in yoga is: *"Where attention goes, energy flows."*

When your attention gets swept up in negative thoughts or habits, you have the conscious ability to recognize them and redirect your focus.

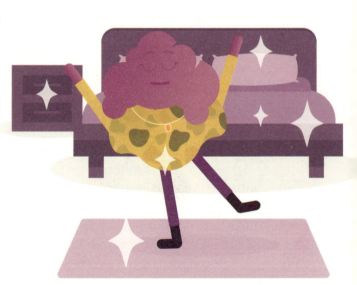

"Yoga is not a religion. It is a science, science of well-being, science of youthfulness, science of integrating body, mind and soul." - Amit Ray

Segment 1: Warm-Up

Full Session Exercise Guide:
habitnest.com/pages/yoga-day-9

1. Seated Torso Circles
30 sec. each direction

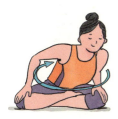

2. Shoulder Socket Rotations
30-60 sec.

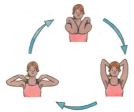

3. Revolved Easy Pose Salute Flow
30-60 sec., alternating

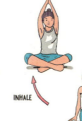

4. Easy Pose Side Bend
30 sec. per side

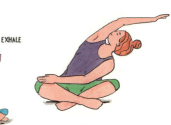

5. Seated Butterfly Pose Wings
30-60 sec.

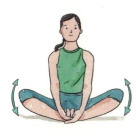

6. Bound Butterfly Wings Flow
30-60 sec.

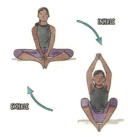

7. Fish Pose w/ Butterfly Legs
60 sec.

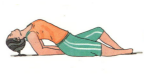

8. Seated Star Pose
60 sec.

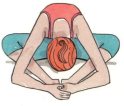

9. Table Top Pose
30 sec.

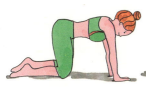

10. Table Top Pose Wrist Stretch
30 sec.

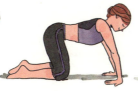

11. Cat-Cow Rib Circles
30-45 sec. each direction

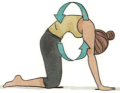

12. Plank Knee-to-Nose Flow
30 sec. per side

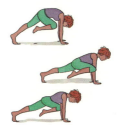

13. Supine Knee Circles
30 sec. each direction

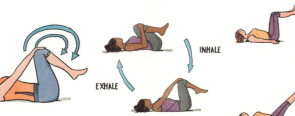

14. Wind Release Flow
30-60 sec.

15. Half Plow Pose Leg Flow
30-60 sec.

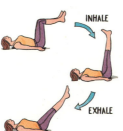

16. Dead Bug Core Workout I
60 sec. alternating

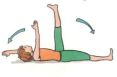
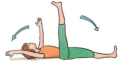

Segment 2: Peak Flow

> Repeat poses 1-8, switching to the opposite side as necessary for asymmetrical poses.

1. Downward-Facing Dog Pose
30 sec.

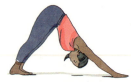

2. Low Lunge Pose
30 sec.

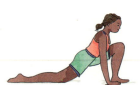

3. High Lunge Pose
30 sec.

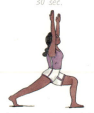

Don't let your left thigh bone drop! Keep it firmly pressed back with pelvis squarely forward.

4. Warrior II Pose
30 sec.

5. Humble Warrior Pose
30 sec.

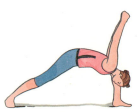

6. Goddess Pose
30-45 sec.

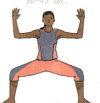

Make sure you tuck your tailbone forward, knit the bottom ribs in, and engage your core.

7. Five-Pointed Star Pose
30 sec.

8. Vinyasa I
30-45 sec.

9. Downward Dog to Mountain Pose Flow
60 sec.

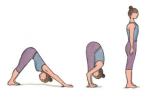

10. Volcano Pose Namaste Salute
30 sec.

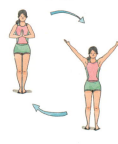

11. Upward Salute to Forward Fold Flow
30-60 sec.

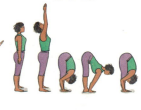

12. Plank Pose
30 sec.

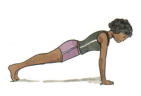

13. Locust Pose
30-60 sec.

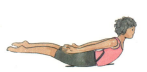

Lift upper body with your sternum, not your chin. The back of the neck should stay long.

14. Thunderbolt Pose
30-60 sec.

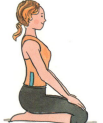

15. Kneeling Pose
30 sec.

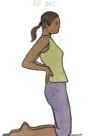

16. Camel Pose
30 sec.

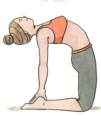

Segment 3: Cool Down

DATE

1. Wind Release Pose
60 sec.

2. Happy Baby Pose
30-60 sec.

3. Supine Spinal Twist II Pose
30 sec. per side

4. Fish Pose
60 sec.

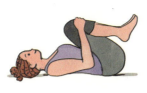
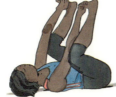
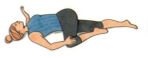
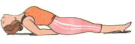

5. Full-Body Stretch Pose
30 sec.

6. Half Plow Pose
30-60 sec.

7. Sage Marichi Pose C
30 sec. per side

8. Sitting Swan Pose
30 sec. per side

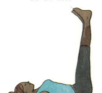
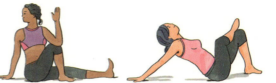

9. Upward-Facing Seated Straddle Pose
30-60 sec.

10. Seated Straddle Forward Fold Pose
30-60 sec.

11. Staff Pose
30 sec.

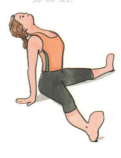
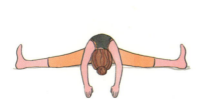
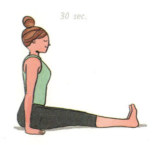

12. Seated Forward Fold Pose
60 sec.

13. Corpse Pose
5 mins

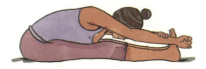
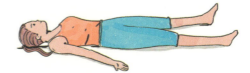

Pro-Tip

Asanas: Listen to your body, focus inward, and stay receptive.

As you continue to build up your yoga practice, it's important to form a deep connection to your body and listen closely to what it's telling you. As you move through your yoga flow, *focus your attention on the sensations in your body.*

Evaluate each sensation... *Does it feel good? Is it painful? Do I feel stable? Is one side stronger or more flexible than the other? Is one muscle tighter than the others?*

If you're feeling any pain beyond the normal burning sensation from exercising, release from the pose immediately and check the steps and alignment cues for the pose.

If it's an alignment issue, it may be a simple fix; however, in some cases, it may just be that your body isn't quite ready for that pose yet. In that case, feel free to skip that pose and pick back up with your flow.

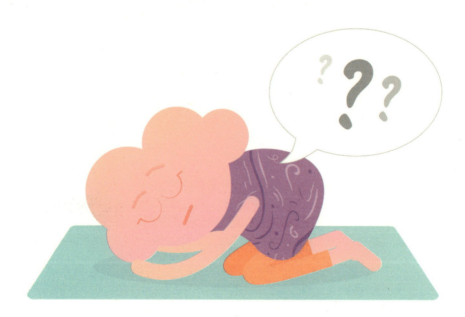

"When you listen to yourself, everything comes naturally. It comes from inside, like a kind of will to do something. Try to be sensitive. That is yoga." - Petri Räisänen

Segment 1: Warm-Up

Full Session Exercise Guide:
habitnest.com/pages/yoga-day-10

1. Easy Pose
30-60 sec.

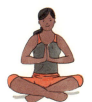

2. Seated Shoulder Rolls
30 sec. forward, then backward

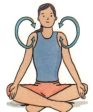

3. Seated Neck Rolls
30 sec. each direction

4. Seated Torso Circles
30 sec. each direction

5. Easy Pose Warm-Up
1-2 mins.

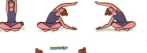
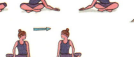

6. Cat-Cow Pose
30-60 sec., alternating

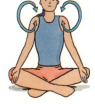

7. Table Top Hip Circles
30-45 sec. each direction

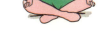

8. Kneeling Sun Salutation
1-2 mins.

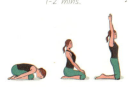

9. Staff Pose
30 sec.

10. Revolved Staff Pose Flow
30-60 sec., alternating

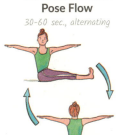

11. Staff Pose Leg Lift & Slide
30 sec. per side

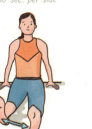

12. Staff Pose Knee Stretch
30 sec. per side

13. Seated Hip Rotations
30 sec. per side

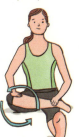

14. Cradle Pose
30 sec. per side

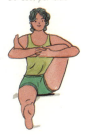

15. Seated Straddle Pose
30-60 sec.

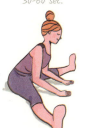

Keep an eye on leg positioning – knees should always be pointing upward to the ceiling.

16. Head-to-Knee Pose
30 sec. per side

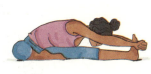

Segment 2: Peak Flow

> Repeat poses 6-12, switching to the opposite side as necessary for asymmetrical poses.

1. Bound Angle Pose
60 sec.

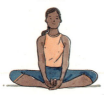

2. Firelog Pose Variation
30 sec. per side

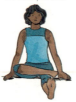

3. Half Cow Face Pose
30 sec. per side

4. Cow Face Pose w/ Eagle Arms
30 sec., then switch arms & legs

5. Mountain Pose
15 sec.

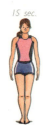

6. Mountain Pose w/ Beginner Eagle Arms
30 sec.

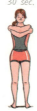

7. Warrior I Pose w/ Eagle Arms
30 sec.

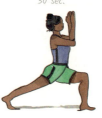

8. Chair Pose w/ Eagle Arms
30 sec.

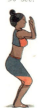

9. Eagle Pose
30 sec.

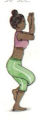

10. Chair Pose w/ Cactus Arms
30 sec.

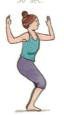

11. Warrior I Pose w/ Cactus Arms
30 sec.

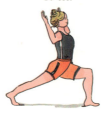

12. Mountain Pose w/ Cactus Arms
30 sec.

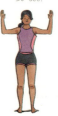

13. Garland Pose
30 sec.

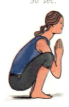

14. Wide Child's Pose
30-60 sec.

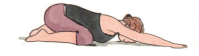

Segment 3: Cool Down

DATE

1. Child's Pose w/ Reverse Prayer
30-60 sec.

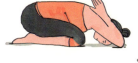

2. Table Top Pose
30 sec.

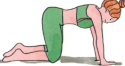

3. Thread the Needle Pose
30-60 sec. per side

4. Staff Pose
30-60 sec.

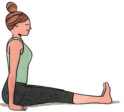

5. Sage Marichi Pose C
30 sec. per side

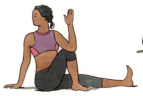

6. Seated Forward Fold
60 sec.

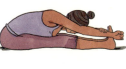

7. Bound Angle Pose
60 sec.

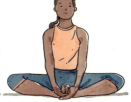

8. Seated Star Pose
60 sec.

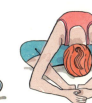

9. Wind Release Pose
60 sec.

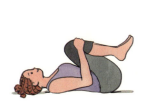

10. Half Plow Pose
30-60 sec.

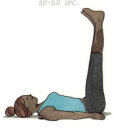

11. Bridge Pose
30-60 sec.

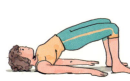

12. Supine Spinal Twist II Pose
30 sec. per side

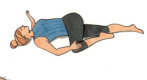

13. Reclining Bound Angle Pose
30-60 sec.

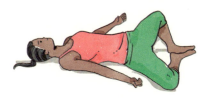

14. Corpse Pose
5 mins.

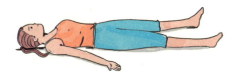

Food for Thought

Pratyahara: the 4 subtypes of Pratyahara.

Pratyahara is essentially a withdrawal of outside stimuli to turn your attention inward.

This detachment from the desires and temptations of our physical/sensory world allows us to take a better look at ourselves and our habits, figure out who we truly are, and pave the way for inner growth.

While Pratyahara plays a similar role as Dharana in that both require getting rid of distractions in order to stay on track and keep our eyes on the prize, there's a key difference between them:

Pratyahara aims more at drawing your attention away from the distractions of everyday life, while Dharana challenges us to direct our attention toward something specific.

Pratyahara can be broken down into 4 types:

- **Indriya Pratyahara** focuses on creating the optimal environment for your mind and body.
- **Prana Pratyahara** is all about controlling and balancing your prana (or universal life energy).
- **Karma Pratyahara** is about your actions and surrendering self-serving motivations, like a personal reward, in favor of acts of kindness and service.
- **Mano Pratyahara** involves withdrawal of the mind from external stimuli, as well as controlling how you act and react to that stimuli.

Practicing this branch of yoga is incredibly helpful for establishing new, positive habits and conquering old, negative habits!

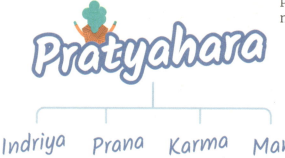

"Yoga allows you to find an inner peace that is not ruffled and riled by the endless stresses and struggles of life." - B.K.S. Iyenga

Segment 1: Warm-Up

Full Session Exercise Guide:
habitnest.com/pages/yoga-day-11

1. Revolved Staff Pose Flow
30-60 sec., alternating

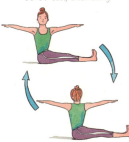

2. Seated Ankle Rotation
30 sec. each direction

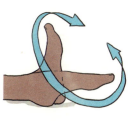

3. Seated Knee Rotation
30 sec. per side

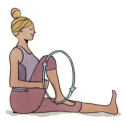

4. Seated Hip Rotation
30 sec. per side

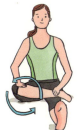

5. Shoulder Socket Rotation
30-60 sec.

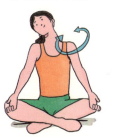

6. Neck Rolls
30 sec. each direction

7. Easy Pose Mudra Flow
30 sec.

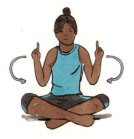

8. Wrist Rolls w/ Hands Clasped
30 sec.

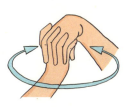

9. Easy Pose Bound Arm Rolls
30 sec. each direction

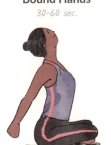

10. Easy Pose w/ Bound Hands
30-60 sec.

11. Easy Pose Forward Fold
30-60 sec.

12. Cat-Cow Rib Circles
30-60 sec.

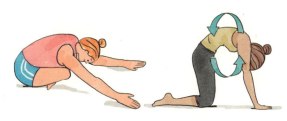

13. Table Top Pose Wrist Stretch
30 sec.

14. Toe Squat
30-60 sec.

15. Thunderbolt Pose Ankle Stretch
30-60 sec.

16. Spinal Rock Pose
30-60 sec.

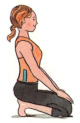
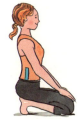
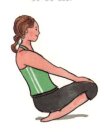

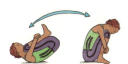

Segment 2: Peak Flow

> Repeat poses 1-8, switching to the opposite side as necessary for asymmetrical poses.

1. Wind Release to Mountain Pose Flow
30-60 sec.

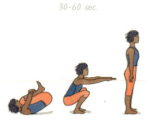

2. Mountain Pose Tiptoes Flow
30 sec.

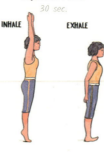

3. Chair Pose
30 sec.

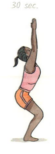

4. Standing Roll-Up Flow
60 sec.

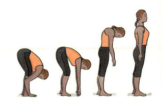

5. Chair to Revolved Chair Pose Flow
30 sec.

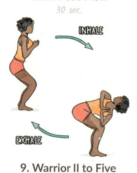

6. Warrior I w/ Cactus Arms Flow
30 sec.

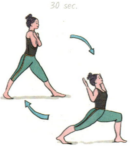

7. Reverse Warrior Pose
30 sec.

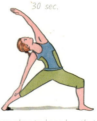

Remember to keep length in the sides of your waist as you enter and hold this pose.

8. Triangle Pose
30 sec.

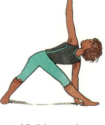

9. Warrior II to Five Pointed Star Flow
60-90 sec.

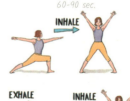

10. Intense Leg Stretch Pose
60 sec.

11. Wide-Legged Forward Fold w/ Ankle Grab
30 sec. per side

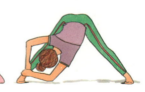

Make sure your thighs stay engaged. Widen the stance if necessary.

12. Mountain Pose Namaste
30 sec.

13. Extended Mountain Pose w/ Hands Interlocked
30 sec.

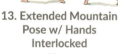

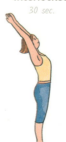

14. Volcano Pose Swan Dive Flow
60 sec.

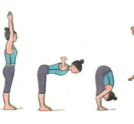

15. Vinyasa II
60 sec.

16. Thunderbolt to Child's Pose Flow
60-90 sec.

Segment 3: Cool Down

DATE

1. Toe Squat
30-60 sec.

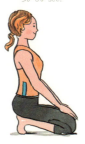

2. Toe Squat w/ Head-to-Knees
30-60 sec.

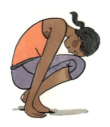

3. Standing Forward Fold
30 sec.

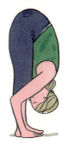

4. Standing Roll-Up Flow
30-60 sec.

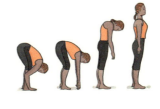

5. Volcano Pose
30 sec.

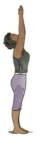

6. Swaying Palm Tree Pose
30 sec. per side

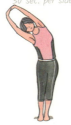

7. Standing Bound Locust Pose
30-60 sec.

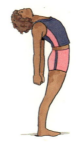

8. Dangling Pose
30-60 sec.

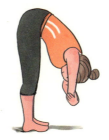

9. Revolved Forward Fold w/ Bent Knee
30 sec. per side

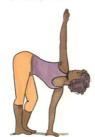

10. Garland Pose
30 sec.

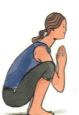

11. Seated Wind Release Pose
60 sec.

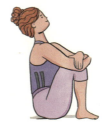

12. Spinal Rock Pose
30-60 sec.

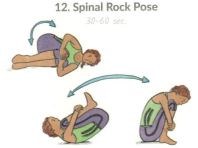

13. Corpse Pose
5 mins.

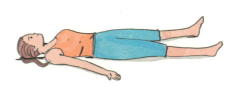

Actionable Challenge

Dharana: Make your mat a sacred space.

If you're finding yourself getting distracted by things you were dealing with before your yoga session started, or things you have to deal with when it's over, you're not alone!

It's a common issue faced by modern Yogis with busy or stressful lives, but you can train your mind to overcome it.

For starters, **make your mat a sacred space.** When you step on the mat, leave everything else behind — all your worries and stresses can wait because this is the time you carved out for yourself and your practice.

While you're on the mat, your only obligation is to yourself.

Before you step onto the mat for your next yoga practice, close your eyes and visualize yourself dropping everything weighing down your mind onto the floor outside the door to your exercise space.

Let yourself feel light and unhindered, take a deep breath, then get started when you're ready.

Bonus: It may also help to change the time of day that you practice.

Something as simple as doing your yoga routine first thing in the morning before starting your day can make a huge difference in limiting internal and external distractions (plus, a peaceful and energizing morning can massively shift your mood for the whole day)!

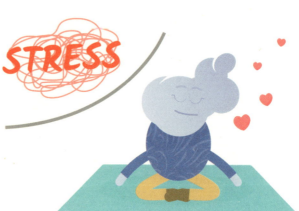

Actionable Challenge Completed: ☐

"You may not be able to control the whole world, but you may learn to control your inner world through yoga." - Debasish Mridha

Segment 1: Warm-Up

Full Session Exercise Guide:
habitnest.com/pages/yoga-day-12

1. Volcano Pose

60 sec.

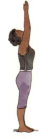

2. Side Lunge

30 sec. per side

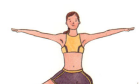

3. Low Lunge w/ Hands to Knee

30 sec. per side

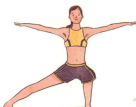

4. Plank to Downward Dog Pose Flow

60 sec.

5. Upward-Facing Dog Pose

60 sec.

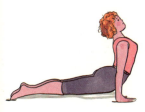

6. Cat-Cow Pose

30-60 sec., alternating

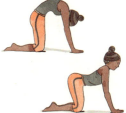

7. Table Top Hip Circles

30-45 sec. each direction

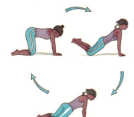

8. Thread the Needle Flow

30 sec. per side

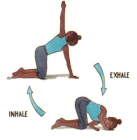

9. Child Pose w/ Arms to One Side

30 sec. per side

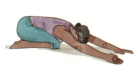

10. Table Top Pose

30 sec.

11. Table Top Pose Wrist Stretch

30 sec.

12. Seated Straddle Pose w/ Windshield Wiper Feet

30-60 sec.

13. Upward-Facing Seated Straddle w/ Toe Grab

30-60 sec.

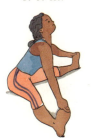

14. Revolved Seated Straddle Pose

30 sec. per side

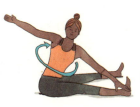

15. Rowing the Boat Flow

30-60 sec.

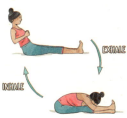

16. Easy Boat Pose w/ Toe Taps

30-60 sec., alternating

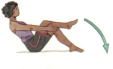
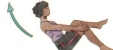

Segment 2: Peak Flow

> Repeat poses 6-12, switching to the opposite side as necessary for asymmetrical poses.

1. Bound Angle Pose
60 sec.
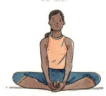

2. Firelog Pose Variation
30 sec. per side
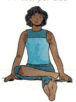

3. Half Cow Face Pose
30 sec. per side

4. Cow Face Pose w/ Eagle Arms
30 sec., then switch arms & legs

5. Mountain Pose
15 sec.
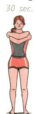

6. Mountain Pose w/ Beginner Eagle Arms
30 sec.

7. Warrior I Pose w/ Eagle Arms
30 sec.
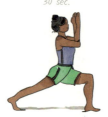

8. Chair Pose w/ Eagle Arms
30 sec.
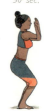

9. Eagle Pose
30 sec.
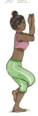

10. Chair Pose w/ Cactus Arms
30 sec.
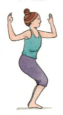

11. Warrior I Pose w/ Cactus Arms
30 sec.
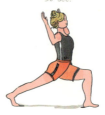

12. Mountain Pose w/ Cactus Arms
30 sec.
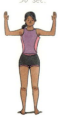

13. Garland Pose
30 sec.
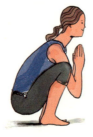

14. Wide Child's Pose
30-60 sec.
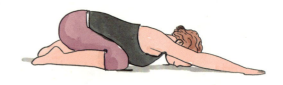

Segment 3: Cool Down

DATE

1. Child's Pose

60 sec.

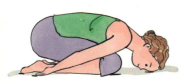

2. Half Lord of the Fishes Pose

60 sec. per side

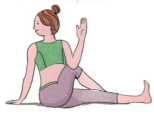

3. Staff Pose w/ Feet Movements

30 sec.

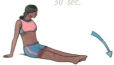
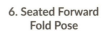

4. Staff Pose w/ Hands Back

15-30 sec.

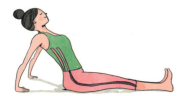

5. Upward Plank Pose

30-60 sec.

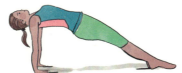

6. Seated Forward Fold Pose

60 sec.

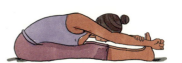

7. Wind Release Pose

60 sec.

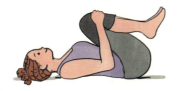

8. Bridge Pose

30-60 sec.

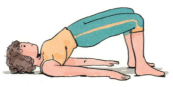

9. Supine Spinal Twist II Pose

30 sec. per side

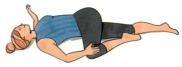

10. Happy Baby Pose

30-60 sec.

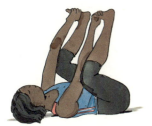

11. Reclining Bound Angle Pose w/ Elbow Grab

30-60 sec.

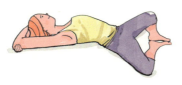

12. Corpse Pose

5 mins.

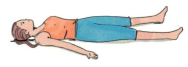

Actionable Challenge

Pranayama: Ocean Breath (Ujjayi).

From the moment our lives begin, our autonomic nervous system (ANS) regulates our breathing, heart rate, and other automatic processes in our bodies.

While we're unable to assume full, conscious control of all other functions regulated by our ANS, we can control our breath; we can turn something that was automatic and unconscious into deliberate and mindful. This, in turn, soothes the rest of the nervous system.

One common breath control method for soothing the nervous system is Ujjayi or Ocean Breath. **This breathing technique is often added to yoga flows - including your flow for today - so give it a shot!**

1. Find a comfortable place to sit. Sit tall and straight with your chin parallel to the floor.
2. Place one hand in your lap and the other in front of your mouth; palm facing you.
3. Open your mouth and exhale into your palm as you would to fog up a mirror. Pay attention to the sound and sensation that is made by your breath when you do this.
4. Now, inhale a breath, making the same sound/sensation.
5. Repeat this for 5-10 cycles, or until you feel like you've gotten the hang of it. Each time, try to inhale for 4 seconds, exhale for 4 seconds.
6. Next, try to create the same sound/sensation, but do so through your nose. Close your mouth on the inhale, and open on the exhale. Repeat for another 5-10 breath cycles, then try it for 5-10 cycles with your mouth open on the inhale and closed on the exhale.
7. When you've gotten the hang of that, it's time to do the actual Ujjayi breathing. Continue breathing through your nose, keeping your mouth closed on both the inhale and exhale.

Remember to breathe with your diaphragm! You may also feel a little self-conscious at first about the sounds, or even struggle to get the hang of it. Just keep practicing and let go of all self-judgment!

Actionable Challenge Completed: ☐

"Meditation brings wisdom; lack of meditation leaves ignorance. Know well what leads you forward and what holds you back, and choose the path that leads to wisdom."
- Buddha

Segment 1: Warm-Up

Full Session Exercise Guide:
habitnest.com/pages/yoga-day-13

1. Ocean Breath
2-3 mins.

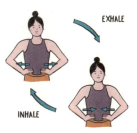

2. Easy Pose
15-30 sec.

3. Seated Torso Circles
30 sec. each direction

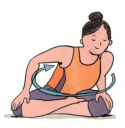

4. Easy Pose Warm-Up
1-2 mins.

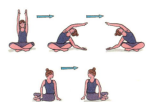

5. Table Top Pose
30 sec.

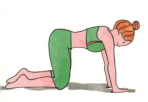

6. Cat-Cow Pose
30-60 sec., alternating

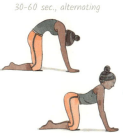

7. Child's Pose
60 sec.

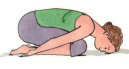

8. Balancing Table Top Pose
30-60 sec. per side

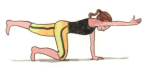

Keep tailbone tucked forward & core engaged. Don't lift arm or leg above shoulder level.

9. Supported Side Plank
30-60 sec. per side

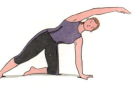

10. Modified Half Gate Pose
30-60 sec. per side

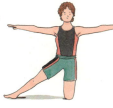

11. Downward-Facing Dog Pose
30-60 sec.

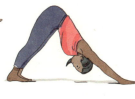

12. Plank Pose
60 sec.

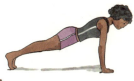

13. Upward-Facing Dog Pose
30 sec.

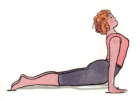

14. Downward-Facing Dog Pose
30 sec.

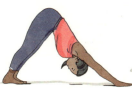

15. Child's Pose
30 sec.

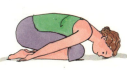

16. Child's Pose Sphinx Flow
30-60 sec.

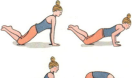

Segment 2: Peak Flow

> Repeat poses 1-15, switching to the opposite side as necessary for asymmetrical poses.

1. Downward Dog to Mountain Pose Flow
~1-2 mins.

2. Chair Pose
30 sec.

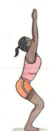

3. Dangling Pose
30-60 sec.

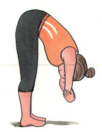

4. Half Forward Fold Pose
20-30 sec.

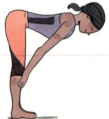

5. Revolved Forward Fold Pose w/ Bent Knee
30 sec.

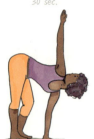

6. Warrior III Leg Sweep Flow
30 sec.

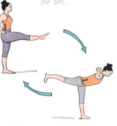

Keep your hips straight and neutral.

7. Standing Wind Release Pose
30 sec.

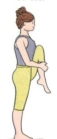

8. High Lunge Pose
30 sec.

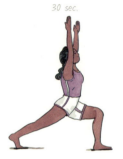

9. Warrior II Pose
30 sec.

10. Reverse Warrior Pose
30 sec.

11. Extended Side Angle Pose
30 sec.

12. Goddess Pose
30-45 sec.

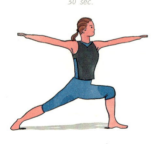

13. Wide-Legged Lateral Squat
30 sec.

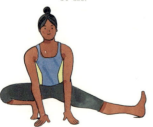

14. Intense Leg Stretch Pose
30 sec.

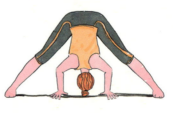

If you're having trouble reaching the floor, try placing your hands on blocks instead.

15. Revolved Wide-Legged Forward Bend Pose
30 sec.

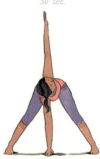

Segment 3: Cool Down

DATE

1. Downward-Facing Dog Pose
30 sec.

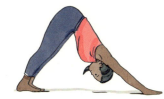

2. Pigeon Pose
30 sec. per side

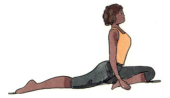

3. Sleeping Swan Pose
30-60 sec. per side

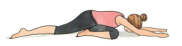

4. Revolved Pigeon Pose
30 sec. per side

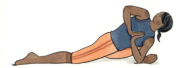

5. Head-to-Knee Pose
30 sec. per side

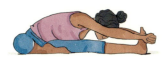

6. Revolved Head-to-Knee Pose
30 sec.

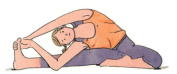

7. Bridge Pose
30-60 sec.

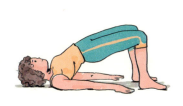

8. One-Legged Bridge Pose
30 sec. per side

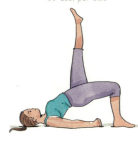

9. Happy Baby Pose
30-60 sec.

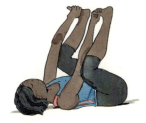

10. Supine Spinal Twist II Pose
30 sec. per side

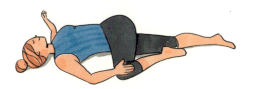

11. Corpse Pose
5 mins.

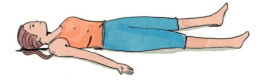

Food for Thought

Dhyana: using yoga as a form of meditative movement.

Meditation is often thought of as something we do while we're physically still and relaxed, but movement can help us to achieve and maintain a meditative state as well.

A meditative state simply boils down to **shifting your consciousness**; and when you're tuning in to your body, focusing your attention inward, and flowing between movements that benefit your body, that's exactly what you're doing!

Many staple poses and flows in yoga, such as the Sun Salutation, are especially helpful for synchronizing the mind, body, and breath in a meditative way.

Yoga isn't the only form of meditative movement - Qigong, Tai Chi, Aikido, and other similar physical practices are all great options as well.

You can even enter a meditative state while going for a walk or run! It's all about learning to tap into that connection between the body and the mind.

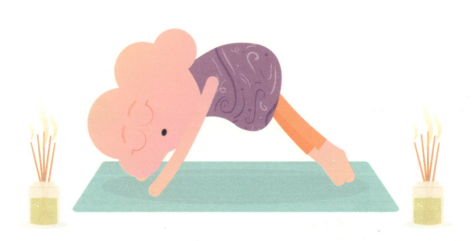

"If you want to conquer the anxiety of life, live in the moment, live in the breath." - Amit Ray

Segment 1: Warm-Up

Full Session Exercise Guide:
habitnest.com/pages/yoga-day-14

1. Volcano Pose
60 sec.

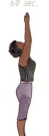

2. Side Lunge
30 sec. per side

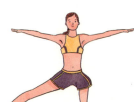

3. Low Lunge w/ Hands to Knee
30 sec. per side

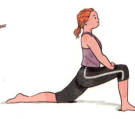

4. Plank to Downward Dog Pose Flow
60 sec.

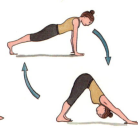

5. Upward-Facing Dog Pose
30 sec.

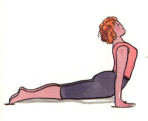

6. Cat-Cow Pose
30-60 sec., alternating

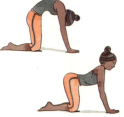

7. Table Top Hip Circles
30-45 sec. each direction

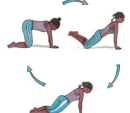

8. Thread the Needle Flow
30 sec. per side

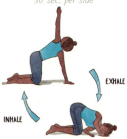

9. Child Pose w/ Arms to One Side
30 sec. per side

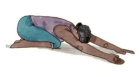

10. Table Top Pose
30 sec.

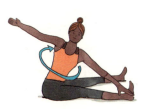

11. Table Top Pose Wrist Stretch
30 sec.

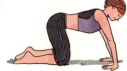

12. Seated Straddle Pose w/ Windshield Wiper Feet
30-60 sec.

13. Upward-Facing Seated Straddle w/ Toe Grab
30-60 sec.

14. Revolved Seated Straddle Pose
30 sec. per side

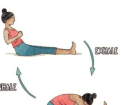

15. Rowing the Boat Flow
30-60 sec.

16. Easy Boat Pose w/ Toe Taps
30-60 sec., alternating

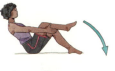
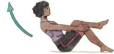

Segment 2: Peak Flow

> Repeat poses 1-8, switching to the opposite side as necessary for asymmetrical poses.

1. Wind Release to Mountain Pose Flow
30-60 sec.

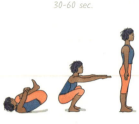

2. Mountain Pose Tiptoes Flow
30 sec.

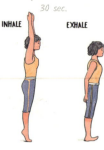

3. Chair Pose
30 sec.

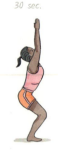

4. Standing Roll-Up Flow
60 sec.

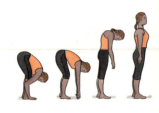

5. Chair to Revolved Chair Pose Flow
30 sec.

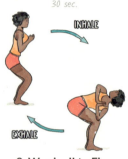

6. Warrior I w/ Cactus Arms Flow
30 sec.

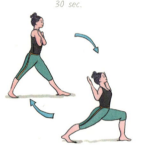

7. Reverse Warrior Pose
30 sec.

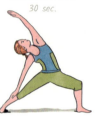

8. Triangle Pose
30 sec.

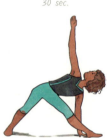

9. Warrior II to Five Pointed Star Flow
60-90 sec.

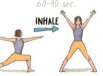
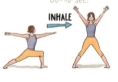

10. Intense Leg Stretch Pose
60 sec.

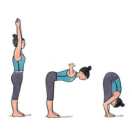

11. Wide-Legged Forward Fold w/ Ankle Grab
30 sec. per side

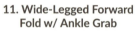
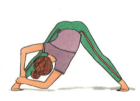

12. Mountain Pose Namaste
30 sec.

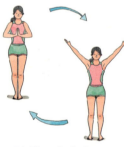

13. Extended Mountain Pose w/ Hands Interlocked
30 sec.

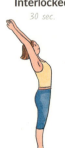

14. Volcano Pose Swan Dive
60 sec.

15. Vinyasa II
60 sec.

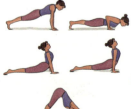

16. Thunderbolt to Child's Pose Flow
60-90 sec.

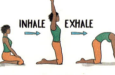

Segment 3: Cool Down

DATE

1. Thread the Needle Pose
30 sec. per side

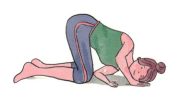

2. Striking Cobra Pose
60 sec.

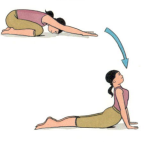

3. Easy Half Bow Pose
30 sec. per side

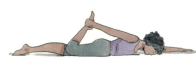

4. Half Wind Release Pose
30 sec. per side

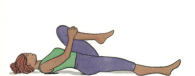

5. Happy Baby Pose
30-60 sec.

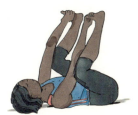

6. Supine Abdominal Twist
30 sec. per side

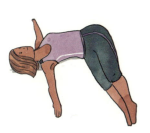

7. Staff Pose
30 sec.

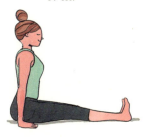

8. Bharadvaja's Twist Pose
30 sec. each side

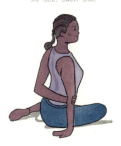

9. Easy Boat Pose
30-60 sec.

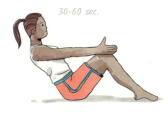

Keep the core and thighs tight and strong to maintain proper balance. Breathe!

10. Upward Plank Pose
30-60 sec.

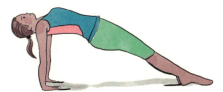

11. Corpse Pose
~5 mins

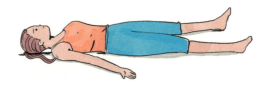

Food for Thought

Chakras: Root Chakra (Muladhara).

In Yoga, the Chakras are a part of our subtle body, meaning we can't see or touch them. Think of them as checkpoints in the body through which all of our spiritual energy flows.

We are all said to have 7 Chakras in our body. Each of them is like a spinning wheel for our energy to flow through that, when unblocked and balanced, work to promote mental, emotional, spiritual, and physical well-being. Each Chakra also has a corresponding color, element, and sound.

The foundation upon which all other Chakras are built upon is the Root Chakra. This Chakra, located at the pelvic floor, controls the basic feelings and instincts at the root of our being; this includes family bonds, core memories, survival instincts, your sense of belonging, and basic human needs (sleep, food, safety, intimacy, etc.)

When your Root Chakra is healthy and balanced, it can help you feel more secure, at ease, grounded, stable, strong, and confident.

When it's blocked or off-balance, however, it can lead to anxiety, low self-esteem, and even self-destructive behavior. Physically, an imbalance may manifest as discomfort or issues in the legs, low back, gut, or bladder.

Properties of this Chakra:

- **Color** - Red
- **Element** - Earth
- **Sound** - Lam

Your Root Chakra can be strengthened and returned to proper balance through certain asanas, such as:

- Wind Release Pose (Pavanmuktasana)
- Head-to-Knee Pose (Janu Sirsasana)
- Lotus Pose (Padmasana)
- Garland Pose (Malasana)

"Each of the seven chakras are governed by spiritual laws, principles of consciousness that we can use to cultivate greater harmony, happiness, and wellbeing in our lives and in the world." - Deepak Chopra

Segment 1: Warm-Up

Full Session Exercise Guide:
habitnest.com/pages/yoga-day-15

1. Constructive Rest Pose w/ Arms Overhead
30-60 sec.

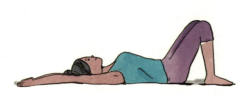

2. Cycling Pose
60-90 sec., alternating legs

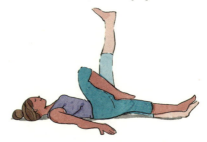

3. Supine Windshield Wipers
30 sec. per side

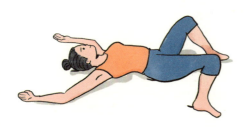

4. Reclined Half Cow Face Pose
30-60 sec. per side

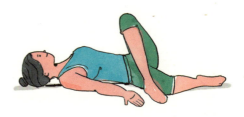

5. Reclined Hand-to-Big-Toe Pose
30 sec. per side

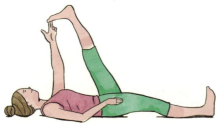

6. Reverse Pigeon Pose
30 sec. per side

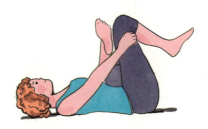

7. Supine Spinal Twist II Pose
30 sec. per side

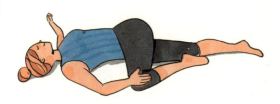

8. Reclined Cow Face Pose
30 sec., then reverse legs & repeat

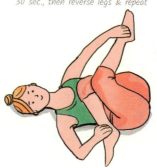

Segment 2: Peak Flow

> Repeat poses 1-15, switching to the opposite side as necessary for asymmetrical poses.

1. Downward Dog to Mountain Pose Flow
1-2 mins.

2. Chair Pose
30 sec.
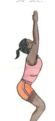

3. Dangling Pose
30-60 sec.
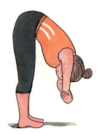

4. Half Forward Fold Pose
15-30 sec.
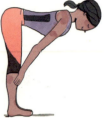

5. Revolved Forward Fold Pose w/ Bent Knee
30 sec.
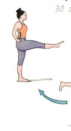

6. Warrior III Leg Sweep Flow
30 sec.
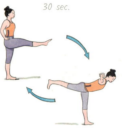

7. Standing Wind Release Pose
30 sec.
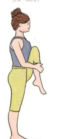

8. High Lunge Pose
30 sec.
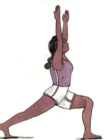

9. Warrior II Pose
30 sec.

10. Reverse Warrior Pose
30 sec.

11. Extended Side Angle Pose
30 sec.

12. Goddess Pose
30-45 sec.

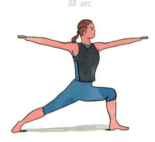

13. Wide-Legged Lateral Squat
30 sec.
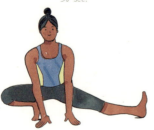

14. Intense Leg Stretch Pose
30 sec.
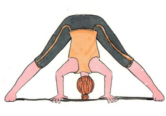

15. Revolved Wide-Legged Forward Bend Pose
30 sec.
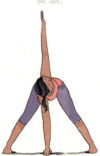

Segment 3: Cool Down

DATE

1. Locust to Wide-Legged Chariot Flow
60-90 sec.

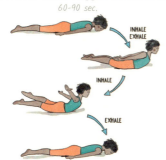

2. Crocodile Pose
30 sec.

3. Downward-Facing Dog Pose
30 sec.

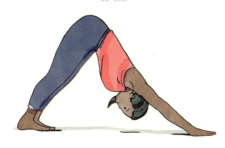

4. Sleeping Swan Pose
30-60 sec. per side

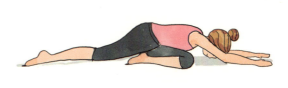

5. Thread the Needle Pose
30 sec. per side

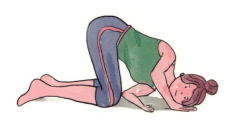

6. Reclined Leg Stretch Flow
30 sec. per side

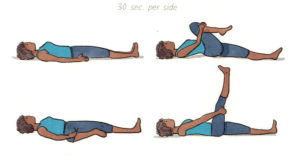

7. Full-Body Stretch to Wind Release Flow
30 sec.

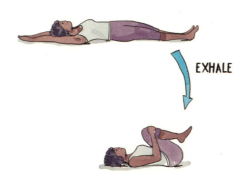

8. Corpse Pose
5 mins

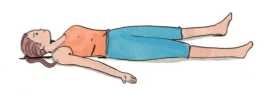

Pro-Tip

Doshas: Kapha.

In Ayurvedic medicine - a holistic practice with Ancient Indian roots - achieving whole-body health requires the balancing of our Doshas.

The 3 Doshas - Kapha, Pitta, and Vata - are said to be the energy centers within us that govern all of our various characteristics, including our personality, emotional traits, and physical appearance.

Mind-body practices, such as your daily yoga routine, are a great way to support a balance between these energies.

Each Dosha comes from combining 2 of the five elements - ether/space, earth, air, water, and fire.

The 2 elements that make up the Kapha Dosha are earth and water, and it's the Dosha in charge of our strength, stability, regulation, patience, growth, and contentment.

You can support and balance this through asanas like:

- Four-Limbed Staff Pose
- Cobra Pose
- Warrior I, II, and III
- Boat Pose
- Standing Forward Fold
- Camel Pose
- Tree Pose
- Pigeon Pose

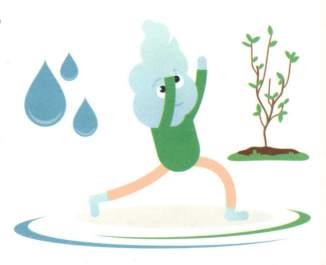

"Yoga is invigoration in relaxation. Freedom in routine. Confidence through self-control. Energy within, and energy without." - Ymber Delecto

Segment 1: Warm-Up

Full Session Exercise Guide:
habitnest.com/pages/yoga-day-16

1. Ocean Breath
2-3 mins.

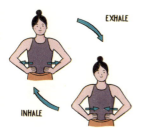

2. Easy Pose
15-30 sec.

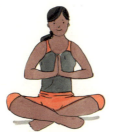

3. Seated Torso Circles
30 sec. each direction

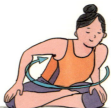

4. Easy Pose Warm-Up
1-2 mins.

5. Table Top Pose
30 sec.

6. Cat-Cow Pose
30-60 sec., alternating

7. Child's Pose
60 sec.

8. Balancing Table Top Pose
30 sec. per side

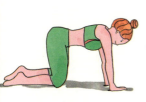
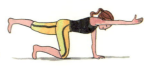

9. Supported Side Plank
30 sec. per side

10. Modified Half Gate Pose
30 sec. per side

11. Downward-Facing Dog Pose
30 sec.

12. Plank Pose
30 sec.

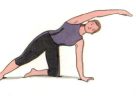
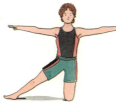
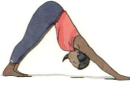
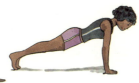

13. Upward-Facing Dog Pose
30 sec.

14. Downward-Facing Dog Pose
30 sec.

15. Child's Pose
30-60 sec.

16. Child's Pose Sphinx Flow
30-60 sec.

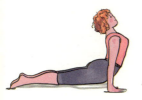
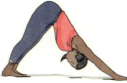
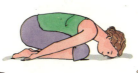
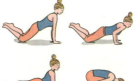

Segment 2: Peak Flow

> Repeat poses 1-8, switching to the opposite side as necessary for asymmetrical poses.

1. Three-Legged Downward-Facing Dog Pose
30 sec.

2. Three-Legged Downward-Facing Dog Pose w/ Knee Rotations
30 sec.
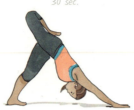

3. Runner's Lunge Pose
30 sec.
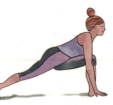

Keep neck neutral or gaze slightly forward. Stack your knee over your ankle.

4. Warrior I Pose
30 sec.
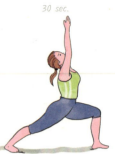

5. Warrior II Pose
30 sec.

6. Reverse Warrior Pose
30 sec.
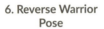

7. Humble Warrior Pose
30 sec.
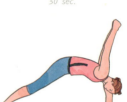

8. Vinyasa I
30 sec.

9. Sphinx Pose
30 sec.

10. Locust Pose
30-60 sec.

11. Easy Half Bow Pose
30 sec. per side

12. Bow Pose
30 sec.

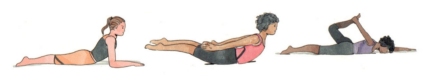

Close eyes and focus on maintaining slow, steady breaths. Release unnecessary tension.

Make sure you're grabbing your feet/ankles from the outside, not the inside.

13. Crocodile Pose
30 sec.

14. Downward Dog Plank Pose Flow
30 sec.

15. Side Plank Pose
30 sec. per side
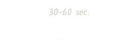

16. Child's Pose
30-60 sec.

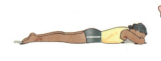
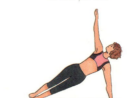
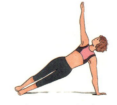

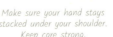

Make sure your hand stays stacked under your shoulder. Keep core strong.

Segment 3: Cool Down

DATE

1. Child's Pose w/ Reverse Prayer
30-60 sec.

2. Table Top Pose
30 sec.

3. Thread the Needle Pose
30-60 sec. per side

4. Staff Pose
30-60 sec.

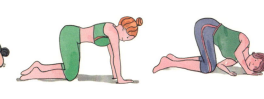
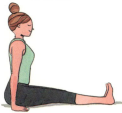

5. Sage Marichi Pose C
30 sec. per side

6. Seated Forward Fold
60 sec.

7. Bound Angle Pose
60 sec.

8. Seated Star Pose
60 sec.

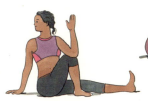
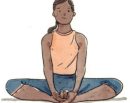
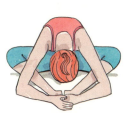

9. Wind Release Pose
60 sec.

10. Half Plow Pose
30-60 sec.

11. Bridge Pose
30-60 sec.

12. Supine Spinal Twist II Pose
30 sec. per side

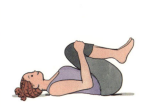
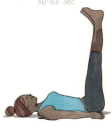
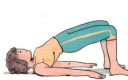
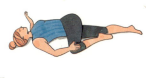

13. Reclining Bound Angle Pose
30-60 sec.

14. Corpse Pose
5 mins.

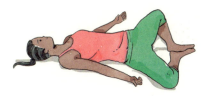
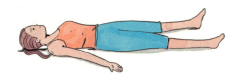

Food for Thought

Koshas: Annamaya.

According to Yoga, there are 5 layers to our individual existence that are called Koshas, which in Sanskrit means "sheaths."

The dense, innermost sheaths are entirely interwoven with and encompassed by the outermost layers, working to promote overall health, encourage inner growth, and deepen your practice.

The first and most dense Kosha is the Annamaya Kosha, which translates to "sheath of food."

That's because this Kosha focuses on your physical body, which is of course fueled by food.

This is an incredibly important sheath because this physical form is how we experience the world around us, how we gather information, and the vehicle by which our thoughts and intentions become actions.

We can take good care of this Kosha simply by taking good care of our bodies - eating healthy, nutritious food, getting exercise (through the asanas, or otherwise!), getting plenty of quality sleep, and taking care of personal hygiene.

Take a moment to consider what your health and fitness goals are, as well as how you can place some extra focus on this Kosha today!

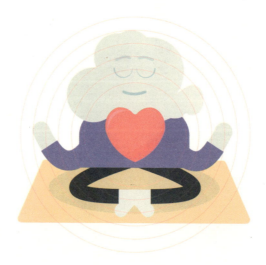

"Take care of your body; it's the only place you have to live." - Jim Rohn

Segment 1: Warm-Up

Full Session Exercise Guide:
habitnest.com/pages/yoga-day-17

1. Easy Pose
30-60 sec.

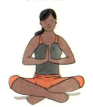

2. Seated Shoulder Rolls
30 sec. forward, then backward

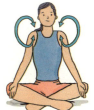

3. Seated Neck Rolls
30 sec. each direction

4. Seated Torso Circles
30 sec. each direction

5. Easy Pose Warm-Up
1-2 mins.

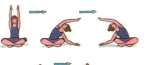

6. Cat-Cow Pose
30-60 sec., alternating

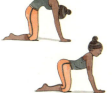

7. Table Top Hip Circles
30-45 sec. each direction

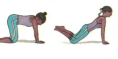
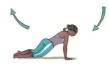

8. Kneeling Sun Salutation
1-2 mins.

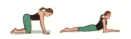

9. Staff Pose
30 sec.

10. Revolved Staff Pose Flow
30-60 sec., alternating

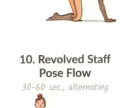

11. Staff Pose Leg Lift & Slide
30 sec. per side

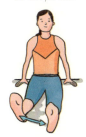

12. Staff Pose Knee Stretch
30 sec. per side

13. Seated Hip Rotations
30 sec. per side

14. Cradle Pose
30 sec. per side

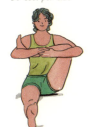

15. Seated Straddle Pose
30-60 sec.

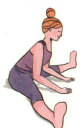

16. Head-to-Knee Pose
30-60 sec. per side

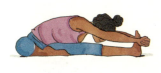

Segment 2: Peak Flow

Repeat poses 1-8, switching to the opposite side as necessary for asymmetrical poses.

1. Three-Legged Downward Dog to Tiger Pose
30 sec.

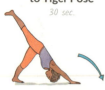

2. Warrior I Pose
30 sec.

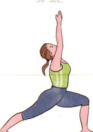

3. Revolved Side Angle Pose
30 sec.

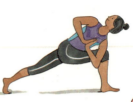

4. Warrior II Pose
30 sec.

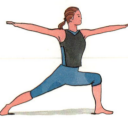

5. Standing Archer Pose
30 sec.

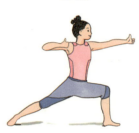

6. Dancing Warrior Pose
30-60 sec.

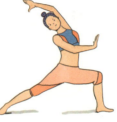

7. Sky Archer Pose
30 sec.

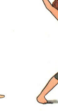

8. Dancer Pose
30 sec.

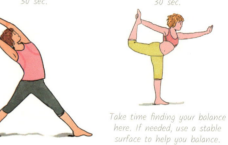

Take time finding your balance here. If needed, use a stable surface to help you balance.

9. Goddess Pose
30-45 sec.

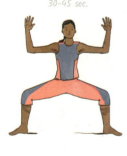

10. Intense Leg Stretch Pose
60 sec.

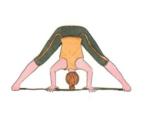

11. Extended Mountain Pose Backbend
30 sec.

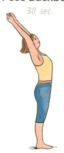

12. Dangling Pose
60 sec.

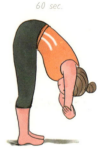

13. Garland Pose
30 sec.

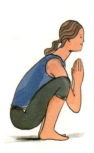

14. Revolved Squat Pose
30 sec. per side

15. Seated Butterfly Pose Wing
30 sec.

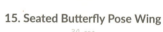

Segment 3: Cool Down

DATE

1. Fish Pose
60 sec.

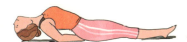

2. Full-Body Stretch Pose
60 sec.

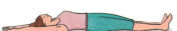

3. Half Wind Release Pose
30 sec. per side

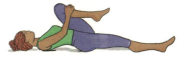

4. Wind Release Pose
60 sec.

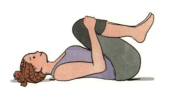

5. Scorpion Twist Pose
30 sec. per side

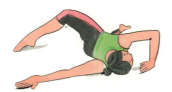

6. Supine Butterfly Pose Wings
30-60 sec.

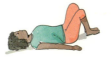
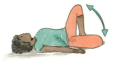

7. Supine Windshield Wipers
30 sec. per side

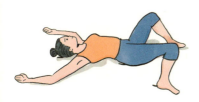

8. Reverse Pigeon Pose
30 sec. per side

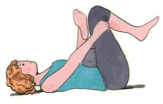

9. Reclined Half Cow Face Pose
30 sec. per side

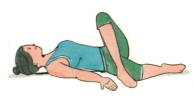

10. Reclined Cow Face Pose
30 sec., then reverse legs & repeat

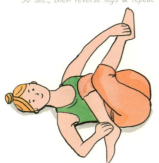

11. Corpse Pose
5 mins.

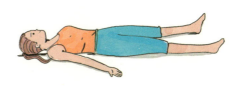

Food for Thought

Yamas: Satya (truthfulness).

The next of the Yamas, Satya, is focused on truthfulness and honesty. Satya requires both restraint and action; restraining yourself from being judgmental or speaking harmfully, and actively making an effort to be more honest with ourselves and others.

Humanity relies on words, both written and spoken, to communicate with and understand each other. We use them to express and define each other, gather and share information, and even change the world. What we say, whether it's to ourselves or someone else, has an impact on our consciousness and mindset.

Right Speech is one main precept of Buddhism that focuses on speaking to ourselves and others in a non-harmful manner and with positive, supportive intentions toward all living beings — a concept very similar to how you would apply both Ahimsa and Satya to your speaking.

Keep in mind that something can be both factually accurate/truthful and harmful at the same time, so balancing Ahimsa and Satya can be a little tricky. These situations have to be evaluated on a case-by-case basis by determining whether or not it's something that's actually necessary to say. For instance, saying that someone's outfit looks silly may be truthful, but that doesn't make it an appropriate practice of Satya.

What it boils down to is this: speak to yourself and others with honesty, kindness, and compassion.

Speak in a way that inspires the best in yourself and others. Practice active listening and look past your initial judgments to see the truth hidden beyond them.

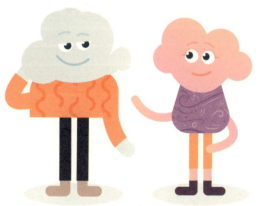

"When you find peace within yourself, you become the kind of person who can live at peace with others." - Peace Pilgrim

Segment 1: Warm-Up

Full Session Exercise Guide:
habitnest.com/pages/yoga-day-18

1. Ocean Breath
2-3 mins.

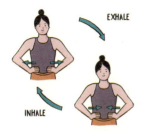

2. Easy Pose
15-30 sec.

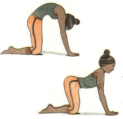

3. Seated Torso Circles
30 sec. each direction

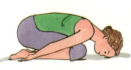

4. Easy Pose Warm-Up
1-2 mins.

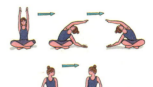

5. Table Top Pose
30 sec.

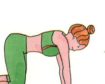

6. Cat-Cow Pose
30-60 sec., alternating

7. Child's Pose
60 sec.

8. Balancing Table Top Pose
30 sec. per side

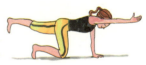

9. Supported Side Plank
30 sec. per side

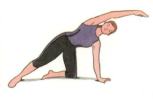

10. Modified Half Gate Pose
30 sec. per side

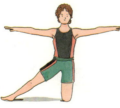

11. Downward-Facing Dog Pose
30 sec.

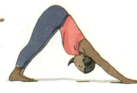

12. Plank Pose
30 sec.

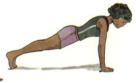

13. Upward-Facing Dog Pose
30 sec.

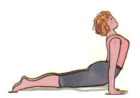

14. Downward-Facing Dog Pose
30 sec.

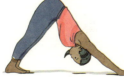

15. Child's Pose
30-60 sec.

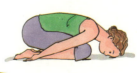

16. Child's Pose Sphinx Flow
30-60 sec.

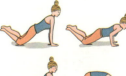
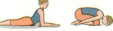

Segment 2: Peak Flow

> Repeat poses 1-7 & 9-12, switching to the opposite side as necessary for asymmetrical poses.

1. Downward-Facing Dog Pose
30 sec.

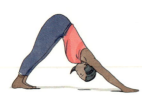

2. Downward Dog Plank Flow
30 sec.

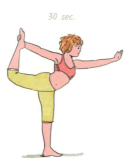

3. Forward Fold Flow
30 sec.

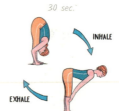

As you transition into Forward Fold Pose, keep spine straight w/o rounding your back.

4. Volcano Pose
30 sec.

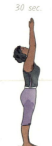

5. Tree Pose
30 sec.

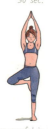

Be very careful in balancing poses like this. Use a stable surface if necessary.

6. Dancer Pose
30 sec.

7. Warrior I Pose
30 sec.

8. Downward Dog to Mountain Pose Flow
30-45 sec.

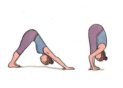

9. Downward-Facing Dog Pose
30 sec.

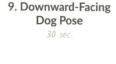

10. Plank Pose
30 sec.

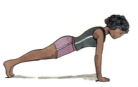

11. Side Plank Pose
30 sec.

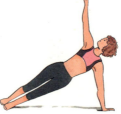

12. Wild Thing Pose
30 sec.

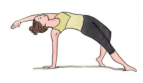

13. Wide Child's Pose
30 sec.

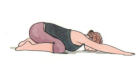

14. Eight-Limbed Striking Cobra Flow
30 sec.

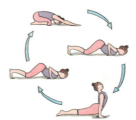

15. Puppy Dog Pose
30-60 sec.

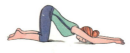

16. Child's Pose
30-60 sec.

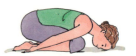

Segment 3: Cool Down

DATE

1. Camel Pose w/ Hands to Floor
30 sec.

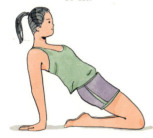

2. Puppy Dog Pose
30-60 sec.

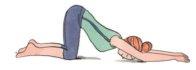

3. Reclined Hero Pose
60 sec.

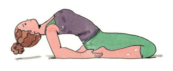

4. Child's Pose
30-60 sec.

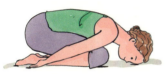

5. Table Top Pose
30-60 sec.

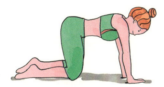

6. Crocodile Pose
30 sec.

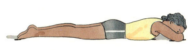

7. Sphinx Pose
60 sec.

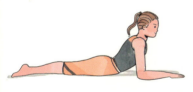

8. Reclining Bound Angle Pose
60 sec.

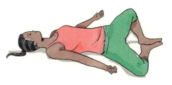

9. Happy Baby Pose
30-60 sec.

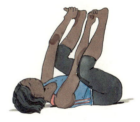

10. Half Wind Release Pose
30 sec. per side

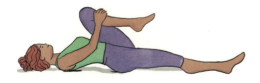

11. Corpse Pose
5 mins.

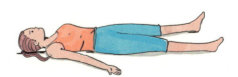

Food for Thought

Niyamas: Santosha (contentment).

Our everyday thoughts are often riddled with thoughts that get in the way of our contentment, such as:

"I'll be happier when I lose weight,"

or

"I'll feel better when I finally get a raise."

Santosha is all about feeling content with yourself, your possessions, and where you're at in life.

It's about appreciating life as it is, while still working toward growth and improvement.

It's great to have goals, desires, and ambitions, but it becomes problematic when your happiness hinges on them.

Don't search for happiness and contentment in the future. Find it in the appreciation of the here and now, right where you are.

If your happiness comes only from external sources, you will always be searching for more; when you search for and cultivate happiness within yourself, you'll never have to wait around for happiness.

During your next yoga practice, challenge yourself to be mindful of your thoughts.

Spend a few moments appreciating yourself, your body (as it is, not as you think it should be!), and your progress thus far.

Remind yourself that you don't have to wait for happiness; you already have everything you need within yourself!

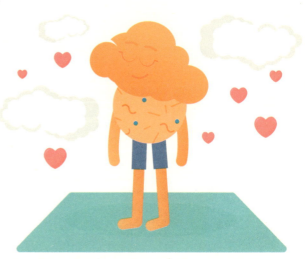

"Happiness is letting go of what you think your life is supposed to look like and celebrating it for everything that it is." - Mandy Hale

Segment 1: Warm-Up

Full Session Exercise Guide:
habitnest.com/pages/yoga-day-19

1. Thunderbolt Pose w/ Torso Twists
60 sec.

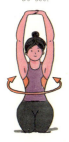

2. Thunderbolt Pose w/ Swinging Arms
30-60 sec.

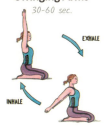

3. Thunderbolt Pose w/ Eagle Arms
30 sec., switch arms & repeat

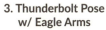
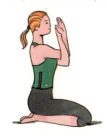

4. Cat-Cow Pose
30-60 sec., alternating

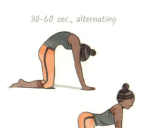

5. Sphinx Pose
60 sec.

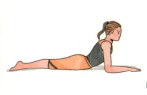

6. Rowing the Boat
30-60 sec.

7. Fish Pose Backbend Flow
60 sec.

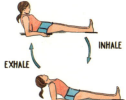
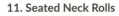

8. Boat Pose Roll-Ups
60 sec.

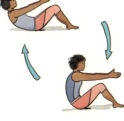

9. Full-Body Stretch to Seated Forward Fold Flow
30-60 sec.

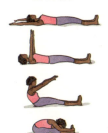

10. Cow Face Pose
30 sec., then switch arms & legs

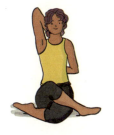

11. Seated Neck Rolls
30 sec. each direction

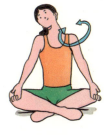

12. Seated Shoulder Rolls
30 sec., forward & backward

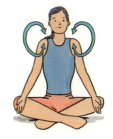

13. Seated Torso Circles
30 sec. each direction

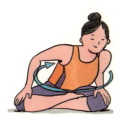

14. Seated Deltoid Stretch
30 sec. per side

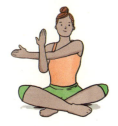

15. Cradle Pose
30 sec. per side

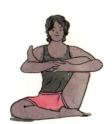

16. Easy Pose Side Bend
30 sec. per side

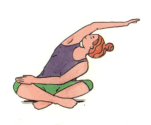

Segment 2: Peak Flow

> Repeat poses 1-4, switching to the opposite side as necessary for asymmetrical poses.

1. Plank to Downward Dog Pose Flow
30 sec.

2. Three-Legged Downward Dog to Tiger Curl Flow
30 sec.

3. Lizard Pose
30-60 sec.

4. Sleeping Swan Pose
30-60 sec.

5. Plank to Downward Dog Pose Flow
30 sec.

6. Standing Forward Fold Pose
30-60 sec.

7. Extended Mountain Pose Backbend
30 sec.

8. Mountain Pose Backbend w/ Cactus Arms
30 sec.

9. Garland Pose w/ Hands Forward
30 sec.

10. Staff Pose
30 sec.

11. Bridge Pose w/ Arm Flow
30-60 sec.

12. Half Plow Pose Flow
30-60 sec.

INHALE
EXHALE

13. Shoulderstand Pose
30-60 sec.

14. Wind Release Pose
60 sec.

Segment 3: Cool Down

DATE

1. Wide Child's Pose
60 sec.

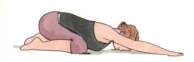

2. Camel Pose w/ Hands to Floor
30 sec.

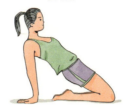

3. Camel Pose
30 sec.

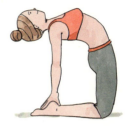

4. Puppy Dog Pose
30-60 sec.

5. Thread the Needle Pose
30 sec. per side

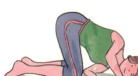

6. Table Top to Child's Pose
30-60 sec.

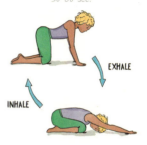

7. Staff Pose
30-60 sec.

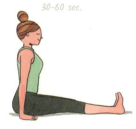

8. Easy Spinal Twist Pose
30 sec. per side

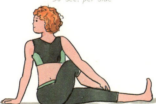

9. Full-Body Stretch Pose
30 sec.

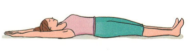

10. Supine Spinal Twist II Pose
30 sec. per side

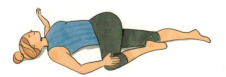

11. Corpse Pose
5 mins.

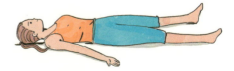

Pro-Tip

Asanas: balance both sides of your body.

The typical yoga routine involves both unilateral (one side of the body) and bilateral (both sides of the body) movement.

Unilateral movements, which are performed on one side and then repeated on the other, can be immensely valuable!

Muscle imbalances, such as tightness or lengthening on one side of the body, can be worsened during bilateral poses and movements because the stronger side attempts to compensate for the weaker side.

Unilateral poses and movements force the weaker, imbalanced sides to pull their own weight, making both sides equal and balanced.

Try to develop an awareness of your unilateral movements.

Pay attention to discrepancies between the two sides, and try to perform the poses the same way on both. This will not only help to deepen your practice, but also prevent injuries and target weaker or imbalanced areas.

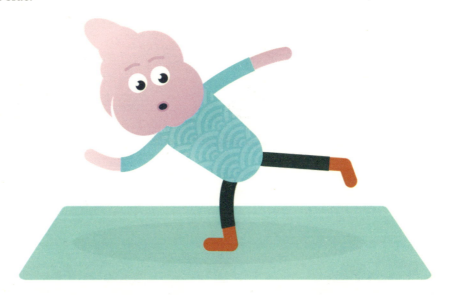

"Balancing in yoga and life is a reflection of our inner state. Can we dance with change? Can we fall and try again with playfulness? Do we have the focus, skill, and attunement to find the still point within it all?" - Shiva Rea

Segment 1: Warm-Up

Full Session Exercise Guide:
habitnest.com/pages/yoga-day-20

1. Supine Arm Sweep I
30-60 sec.

Keep your shoulder blades planted firmly on the floor/mat throughout these movements.

2. Supine Arm Sweep II
30-60 sec.

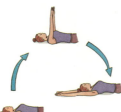

3. Half Wind Release Pose
30-60 sec. per side

4. Dead Bug Core Exercise II
~2 mins.

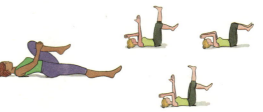

5. Staff Pose
30 sec.

6. Seated Forward Fold Pose
60 sec.

7. Staff Pose Knee Stretches
30 sec. per side

8. Half Lord of the Fishes Pose
30 sec. per side

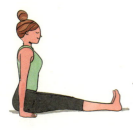

9. Cradle Pose
30 sec. per side

10. Seated Neck Rolls
30 sec. each direction

11. Wrist Rolls w/ Clasped Hands
30 sec.

12. Cat-Cow Pose
30-60 sec., alternating

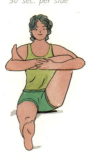
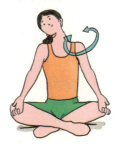
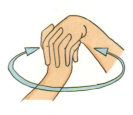
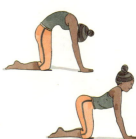

13. Balancing Table Top Knee-to-Nose Crunches
30 sec. per side

14. Child's Pose
30 sec.

15. Simple Grounded Shakti Flow
~2 mins.

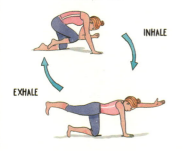
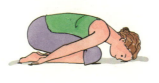
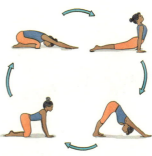

Segment 2: Peak Flow

> Repeat poses 1-15, switching to the opposite side as necessary for asymmetrical poses.

1. Downward Dog to Mountain Pose Flow
60-90 sec.

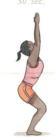

2. Chair Pose
30 sec.

3. Dangling Pose
30-60 sec.

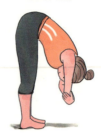

4. Half Forward Fold Pose
20-30 sec.

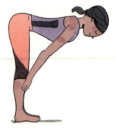

5. Revolved Forward Fold Pose w/ Bent Knee
30 sec.

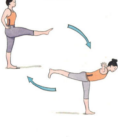

6. Warrior III Leg Sweep Flow
30 sec.

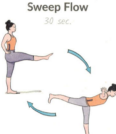

7. Standing Wind Release Pose
30 sec.

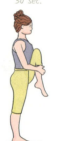

8. High Lunge Pose
30 sec.

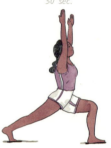

9. Warrior II Pose
30 sec.

10. Reverse Warrior Pose
30 sec.

11. Extended Side Angle Pose
30 sec.

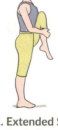

12. Goddess Pose
30-45 sec.

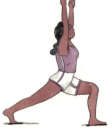

13. Wide-Legged Lateral Squat
30 sec.

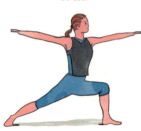

14. Intense Leg Stretch Pose
30 sec.

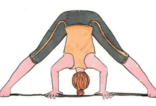

15. Revolved Wide-Legged Forward Bend Pose
30 sec.

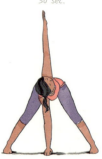

Segment 3: Cool Down

DATE

1. Thunderbolt Pose Salute
60 sec.

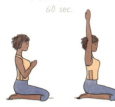

2. Puppy Dog Pose
30-60 sec.

3. Staff Pose
30 sec.

4. Seated Forward Fold Pose
60 sec.

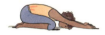

5. Sitting Swan Pose
30 sec. per side

6. Upward-Facing Seated Straddle Pose
30-60 sec.

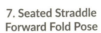

7. Seated Straddle Forward Fold Pose
30-60 sec.

8. Cosmic Egg Pose
30-60 sec.

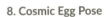

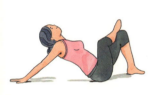
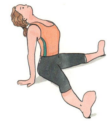
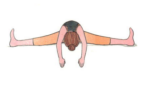
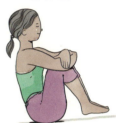

9. Happy Baby Pose
30-60 sec.

10. Reclining Bound Angle Pose w/ Elbow Grab
30-60 sec.

11. Constructive Rest Pose
30-60 sec.

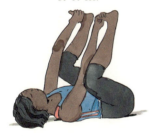
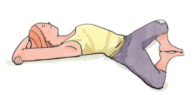
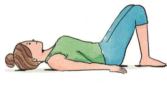

12. Supine Spinal Twist Pose
30 sec. per side

13. Corpse Pose
5 mins.

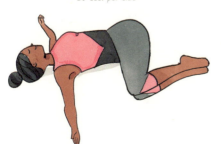
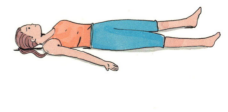

Pro-Tip

Dharana: Choosing a good outdoor spot to practice.

Moving your practice outdoors occasionally is a great way to elevate your yoga practice.

Exercising outdoors is proven to:

- Boost your mood, mental health, and self-esteem.
- Relieve symptoms of stress and anxiety.
- Stimulate and engage your mind and senses.
- Lead to an increase in calories burned, due to the change in environment distracting you from how tired your muscles are.
- Challenge your body by forcing it to adapt to a different temperature, humidity, and environment than you're used to.

Even if you don't leave your porch or backyard, consider moving your yoga practice outdoors for a day to see how it feels!

Yoga can technically be performed anywhere — all you need is your mind and body!

Nonetheless, there are a few factors to keep in mind when choosing an outdoor spot:

- **Your physical limitations** — If completing your routine outdoors would be too challenging or uncomfortable, don't push yourself to do it! This journey is all about finding what feels right to you and your body.
- **The weather/temperature outside** — It's best to practice in fair weather, when it's not too hot or cold. Don't put yourself at risk by trying to exercise in potentially unsafe conditions.
- **Shade** — Try to pick a spot with plenty of shade so that the sun isn't shining directly on you or in your eyes.
- **Ground** — Choose a spot that provides you plenty of relatively flat and level ground space to move around. Clear away any sharp sticks, plants, rocks, or objects.
- **The view** — While a gorgeous view isn't necessary, it definitely helps!

If you don't have a good space to practice directly outside your home (such as the porch, balcony, or backyard), you could try going to a nearby beach, lake, hiking trail, or park!

"The most important pieces of equipment you need for doing yoga are your body and mind." - Rodney Yee

Segment 1: Warm-Up

Full Session Exercise Guide:
habitnest.com/pages/yoga-day-21

1. Thunderbolt Pose
30-60 sec.

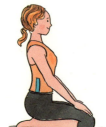

2. Revolved Thunderbolt Pose
30 sec. per side

3. Kneeling Side Bends
30 sec. per side

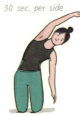

If you can't reach the floor in this pose, try placing your hand on a block instead!

4. Cat-Cow Pose
30-60 sec., alternating

5. Child's Pose Sphinx Flow
60-90 sec.

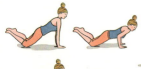

6. Wide Child's Pose
30 sec.

7. Wide-Legged Vinyasa Flow
30-60 sec.

8. Downward Dog to Mountain Pose Flow
30 sec.

9. Mountain Pose Tiptoes Flow
30 sec.

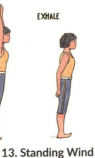

INHALE   EXHALE

10. Standing Arm Circles
30 sec. forward & backward

11. Easy Joint Warm-Up Flow
2-3 mins.

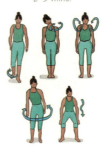

12. Mountain Pose Forward Fold Arm Swings
30 sec.

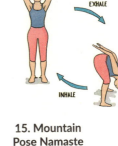

EXHALE

INHALE

13. Standing Wind Release Pose
30 sec. per side

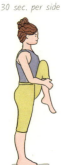

14. Standing Quad Stretch
30 sec. per side

15. Mountain Pose Namaste
30 sec.

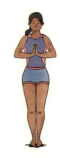

Segment 2: Peak Flow

> Repeat poses 1-8, switching to the opposite side as necessary for asymmetrical poses.

1. Mountain Pose
30 sec.

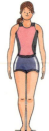

2. One-Legged Mountain Pose w/ Side Bend
30 sec.

3. Chair Pose
30 sec.

4. Revolved Chair Pose
30 sec.

5. Vinyasa I
30 sec.

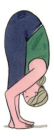

6. Reverse Warrior Pose
30 sec.

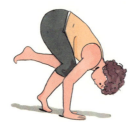

7. Twisted Reverse Warrior Pose
30 sec.

8. Extended Side Angle Pose
30 sec.

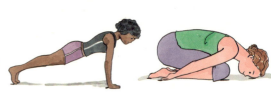

9. Standing Forward Fold Pose
30-60 sec.

10. Crow Pose w/ Toe Taps
30 sec. each side

11. Plank Pose
30 sec.

12. Child's Pose
30-60 sec.

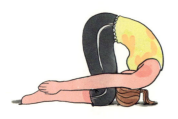

13. Rabbit Pose
30-60 sec.

14. Toe Squat Pose w/ Cat-Cow Flow
30-60 sec.

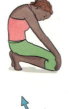
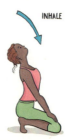

INHALE

EXHALE

15. Thunderbolt Pose Heart Opener
60 sec.

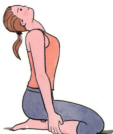

Segment 3: Cool Down

DATE

1. **Wind Release Pose**
   60 sec.

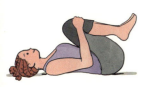

2. **Happy Baby Pose**
   30-60 sec.

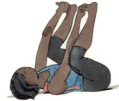

3. **Supine Spinal Twist II Pose**
   30 sec. per side

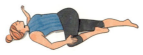

4. **Fish Pose**
   60 sec.

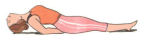

5. **Full-Body Stretch Pose**
   30-60 sec.

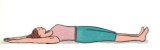

6. **Half Plow Pose**
   30-60 sec.

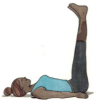

7. **Sage Marichi Pose C**
   30 sec. per side

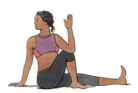

8. **Sitting Swan Pose**
   30 sec. per side

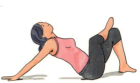

9. **Upward-Facing Seated Straddle Pose**
   30-60 sec.

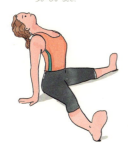

10. **Seated Straddle Forward Fold Pose**
    30-60 sec.

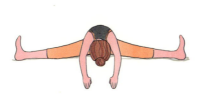

11. **Staff Pose**
    30 sec.

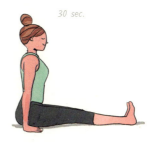

12. **Seated Forward Fold Pose**
    60 sec.

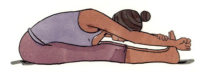

13. **Corpse Pose**
    5 mins.

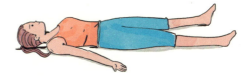

Recap Questions

1. What elements of my practice have I found to be the most beneficial? Why?

2. What have I learned about myself through my practice so far? About who I am and who I'm growing into and aim to be?

3. What poses (if any) have I struggled the most with? What is the root cause of that struggle (i.e. a tight muscle making it hard to get into the pose), and how can I address it?

4. How have my daily habits changed since beginning this practice? What habits hinder my practice, and how can I address them?

5. How has this practice helped me cultivate a better mindset that I can carry into other aspects of life?

Phase 2 Done.

Phase 3: Flow 22 - 66

Rewiring Your Brain

My main yoga goal for this phase:

Phase 2 Overview

Can you believe how far you've come since beginning this journey?! Well, believe it! You made it, and you should be proud of yourself for already completing 21 intense yoga flows.

By now, you've likely noticed that yoga transforms your mind as much as (if not more than) it transforms your body. It illuminates everything within you, shining bright even in the areas of yourself that you didn't even notice. Embrace it and keep growing!

This phase serves to truly integrate and cement this practice into your life.

Keep showing up to the mat daily, and keep applying what you learn about yoga and yourself to your everyday life.

This is the perfect time to start experimenting with new poses, meditations, and breathing techniques to deepen your practice and find what works for you!

Let's go, let's grow!

Takeaways from this phase

❖ Deepen your study of the yogic sutras & principles.

❖ Try a few new things along the way to expand & diversify your practice.

❖ Extended consistency throughout this phase ensures that your practice truly becomes a habit.

❖ Celebrate your amazing progress!

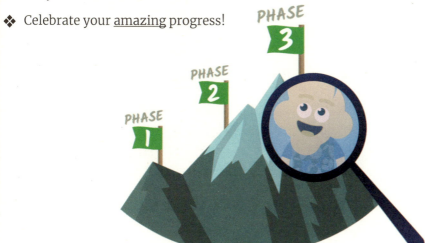

Actionable Challenge

Pranayama: Alternate Nostril Breathing.

Alternate Nostril Breathing (ANB) is the perfect tool for soothing your mind and body.

Otherwise known as Nadi Shodhana, this technique is a favorite for many Yogis and non-Yogis alike. It balances the flow of air, quiets your mind, and eliminates racing thoughts.

Try this Alternate Nostril Breathing Method in a stressful or anxious moment:

1. Find somewhere comfortable to sit. Keep your spine straight and tall, and your chest open.
2. Relax your left hand in your lap, and bring your right hand in front of your face.
3. Rest the index and middle fingers of your right hand gently in the space between your eyebrows. There's no need to apply any pressure, just lightly anchor them there.
4. Take a deep breath through your nose, taking a moment to prepare yourself.
5. With your right thumb, close your right nostril. Take a slow, steady inhale, and at the top of the inhale, use your ring finger to close your left nostril as well.
6. Hold the breath with both nostrils closed for a few moments, then open your right nostril for a steady exhale.
7. Inhale again through the right nostril and hold it for a few moments, plugging both nostrils, then open your left nostril and exhale slowly.
8. Inhale once more through your left nostril, plugging both at the top, then exhaling through the right nostril
9. Repeat this for 5-10 more breath cycles, trying to keep your timing consistent. Try inhaling for 4 counts, holding for 4 counts, and exhaling for 4 counts, then slowly working up to slightly longer counts.

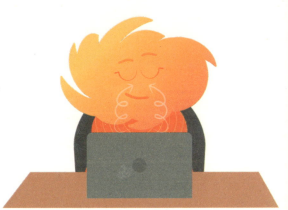

Actionable Challenge Completed: ☐

"Sometimes the most important thing in a whole day is the rest we take between two deep breaths." - Etty Hillesum

Segment 1: Warm-Up

Full Session Exercise Guide:
habitnest.com/pages/yoga-day-22

1. Alternate Nostril Breathing
2 mins.

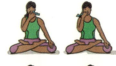

2. Easy Pose Warm-Up
1-2 mins.

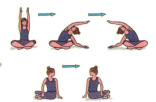

3. Seated Neck Rolls
30 sec. each direction

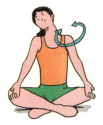

4. Neck Twists
30-60 sec., alternating

5. Side-to-Side Neck Stretch
30 sec. per side

6. Forward-to-Backward Neck Stretch
30 sec. forward & backward

7. Cat-Cow Pose w/ Lateral Leg Extension
30 sec. per side

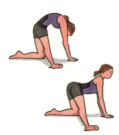

8. Tiger Pose Crunches
30 sec. per side

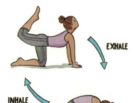

9. Table Top Pose Wrist Stretch
30 sec.

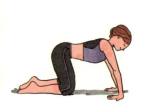

10. Child's Pose Cat-Cow Flow
60 sec.

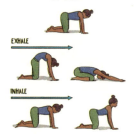

11. Thread the Needle Pose Flow
30 sec. per side

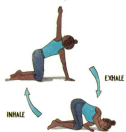

12. Dolphin to Downward Dog Push-Ups
30-60 sec.

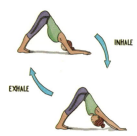

13. Half Headstand Pose
30-60 sec.

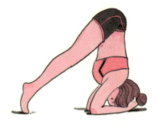

14. Tripod Pose Prep
30 sec. per side

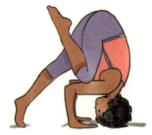

15. Crocodile Pose on Elbows
30 sec.

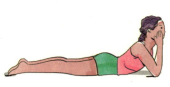

Segment 2: Peak Flow

> Repeat poses 1-8, switching to the opposite side as necessary for asymmetrical poses.

1. Three-Legged Downward-Facing Dog Pose
30 sec.

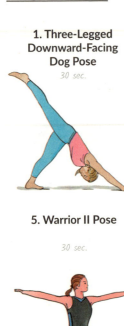

2. Three-Legged Downward-Facing Dog Pose w/ Knee Rotations
30 sec.

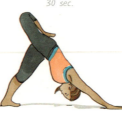

3. Runner's Lunge Pose
30 sec.

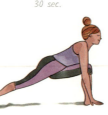

4. Warrior I Pose
30 sec.

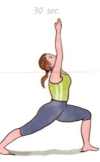

5. Warrior II Pose
30 sec.

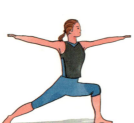

6. Reverse Warrior Pose
30 sec.

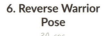

7. Humble Warrior Pose
30 sec.

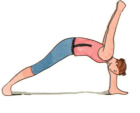

8. Vinyasa I
30 sec.

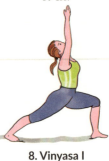

9. Sphinx Pose
30 sec.

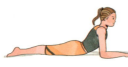

10. Locust Pose
30 sec.

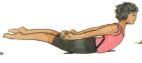

11. Easy Half Bow Pose
30 sec. per side

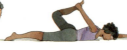

12. Bow Pose
30 sec.

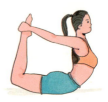

13. Crocodile Pose
30 sec.

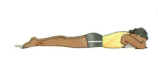

14. Downward Dog Plank Pose Flow
30 sec.

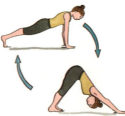

15. Side Plank Pose
30 sec. per side

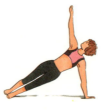

16. Child's Pose
30-60 sec.

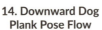

Segment 3: Cool Down

DATE

1. Child's Pose w/ Reverse Prayer
30-60 sec.

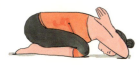

2. Table Top Pose
30 sec.

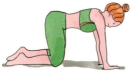

3. Thread the Needle Pose
30 sec. per side

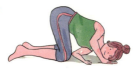

4. Staff Pose
30-60 sec.

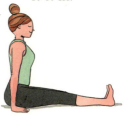

5. Sage Marichi Pose C
30 sec. per side

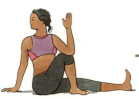

6. Seated Forward Fold
60 sec.

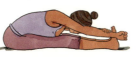

7. Bound Angle Pose
60 sec.

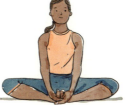

8. Seated Star Pose
60 sec.

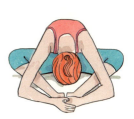

9. Wind Release Pose
60 sec.

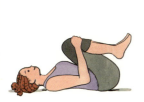

10. Half Plow Pose
30-60 sec.

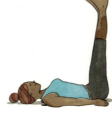

11. Bridge Pose
30-60 sec.

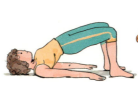

12. Supine Spinal Twist II Pose
30 sec. per side

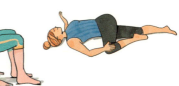

13. Reclining Bound Angle Pose
30-60 sec.

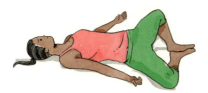

14. Corpse Pose
5 mins.

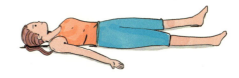

Food for Thought

Dharana: be in the here & now.

As you progress through this journey of building a yoga practice, you'll inevitably encounter some frustration with yourself for not being better at certain things, or struggling with any elements of your practice.

Though these thoughts are inevitable, you can't allow them to overtake your practice and distract you from progress and growth.

You're not going to be amazing at everything in your practice right off the bat - and that's okay! Embrace it and use it as a learning opportunity!

Don't worry about what happened yesterday or what might happen tomorrow; just be present where you are.

Everyone starts as a beginner, and each person's practice is as unique as they are.

Developing a yoga practice isn't about being the best meditator or mastering the hardest asanas; It's about doing the best you can for yourself and those around you.

You're not in competition with anyone. You're not trying to be better than anyone else but yourself, and the only way to make that change is to become aware of who you are in the present moment and steer that awareness toward progress.

Be present wherever you are on this journey.

You are already whole, capable, and full of possibilities, but you can't unlock that if your focus is anywhere but the present! The fact that you've made it this far is an accomplishment in itself.

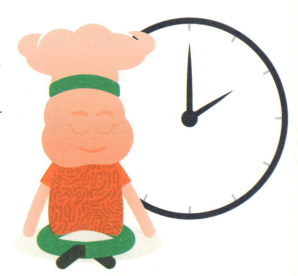

"Yoga takes you into the present moment. The only place where life exists."
- Patañjali

Segment 1: Warm-Up

Full Session Exercise Guide:
habitnest.com/pages/yoga-day-23

1. Bound Angle Pose
60 sec.

2. Cradle Pose
30 sec. per side

3. Head-to-Knee Pose
30 sec. per side

4. Revolved Head-to-Knee Pose
30 sec. per side

5. Crocodile Pose
30 sec.

6. Locust Pose
30-60 sec.

7. Dolphin Pose
60 sec.

8. Three-Legged Downward-Facing Dog Pose
30 sec. per side

9. Lizard Pose
30-60 sec. per side

10. Triangle Pose w/ Bent Knee
30 sec. per side

11. Standing Forward Fold Pose
30 sec.

12. Dangling Pose
30 sec.

13. Chair Pose
30 sec.

14. Standing Backbend Pose
30-60 sec.

Repeat poses 8-10, switching to the opposite side as necessary for asymmetrical poses.

Segment 2: Peak Flow

> Repeat poses 1-8, switching to the opposite side as necessary for asymmetrical poses.

1. Downward-Facing Dog Pose
30 sec.

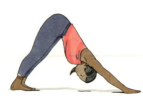

2. Garland Pose
30 sec.

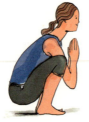

3. Twisted Dragon Pose
30 sec.

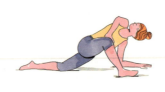

4. Twisted Low Lunge Pose
30 sec.

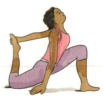

If the twist in this pose is too much for you, grab the raised foot with the matching hand.

5. Warrior I Pose
30 sec.

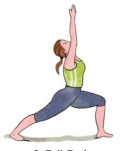

6. Reverse Warrior Pose
30 sec.

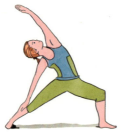

7. Goddess Pose
30-45 sec.

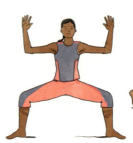

8. Plank Pose
30 sec.

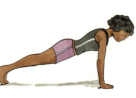

9. Full-Body Stretch Pose
30 sec.

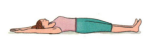

10. Half Boat Pose
30-60 sec.

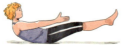

Use your outstretched arms to help hold the shoulders and chest in alignment.

11. Constructive Rest Pose
30-60 sec.

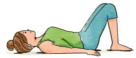

12. Bridge Pose w/ Arm Flow
30-60 sec.

13. Supine Spinal Twist Pose
30 sec. per side

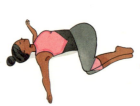

14. Reclined Hand-to-Big-Toe Pose
30 sec. per side

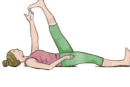

15. Happy Baby Pose
30-60 sec.

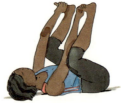

16. Reclining Bound Angle Pose
30-60 sec.

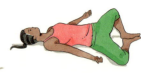

Segment 3: Cool Down

DATE

1. Child's Pose

1-2 mins.

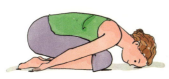

Take your time here to really rest, relax, and ground yourself.

2. Cobra Pose

30-60 sec.

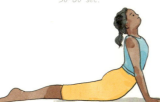

3. Plank Pose

30 sec.

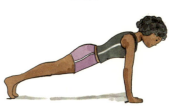

4. Downward-Facing Dog Pose

30 sec.

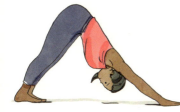

5. Table Top Pose

30 sec.

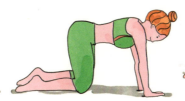

6. Puppy Dog Pose

30-60 sec.

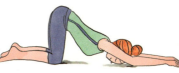

7. Puppy Dog Pose Neck Stretch

30 sec. per side

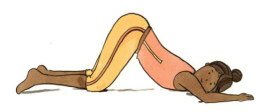

8. Revolved Puppy Dog Pose

30 sec. per side

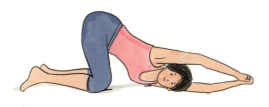

9. Half Wind Release Pose

30 sec. per side

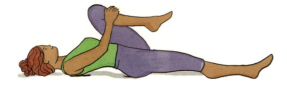

10. Corpse Pose

5 mins.

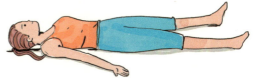

Pro-Tip

Dhyana: play soothing music or ambient noise during your practice.

Music has a profound impact on our mind and body, but does it pair well with yoga and meditation?

The decision to incorporate music with your flow is completely based on personal preference.

Some find music or ambient noise distracting, while others find that it helps them reach and maintain a deeper meditative state.

Give it a try for yourself and see if music can be a valuable addition to your practice!

It's best to pick slow, soothing instrumentals or noises (such as the sound of rain, ocean waves, or white noise).

Keep the volume low, and feel free to turn it off if you find that it's too distracting!

If you choose to add music or ambient noise to your practice, try to choose audio that:

- Doesn't involve any singing/talking, which can be highly distracting
- Isn't too fast, loud, or stimulating
- Doesn't evoke strong emotions

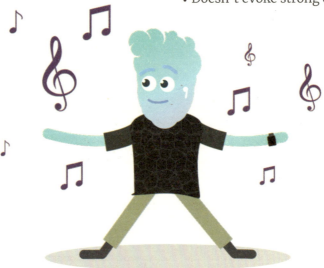

"Yoga is like music: the rhythm of the body, the melody of the mind, and the harmony of the soul create the symphony of life." - B.K.S. Iyengar

Segment 1: Warm-Up

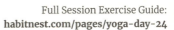

1. Easy Pose
30-60 sec.

2. Easy Pose Warm-Up
1-2 mins.

3. Cat-Cow to Child's Pose Flow
1-2 mins.

4. Thread the Needle Flow
30 sec. per side

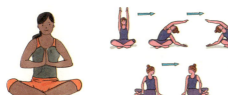
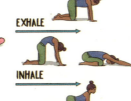
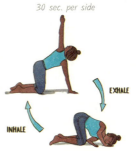

5. Table Top Pose w/ Leg Raise
30 sec. per side

6. Supported Side Plank
30 sec. per side

7. Low Lunge w/ Hands to Knee
30 sec. per side

8. One-Legged Bow Pose
30 sec. per side

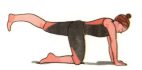
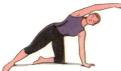
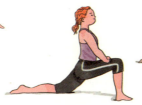
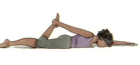
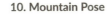

9. Vinyasa I
30 sec.

10. Mountain Pose
30 sec.

11. Standing Wind Release Pose
30 sec. per side

12. Mountain Pose w/ Twist
30 sec. per side

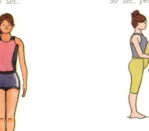
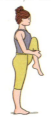

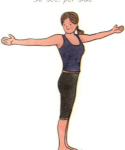

13. Standing Backbend Pose
30-60 sec.

14. Standing Forward Fold w/ Knees Bent
30-60 sec.

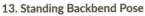
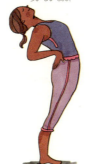
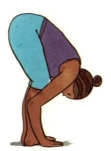

Segment 2: Peak Flow

> Repeat poses 1-12, switching to the opposite side as necessary for asymmetrical poses.

1. Five-Pointed Star Pose
30 sec.

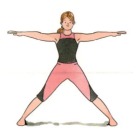

2. Triangle Pose
30 sec.

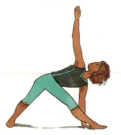

3. Revolved Triangle Pose
30 sec.

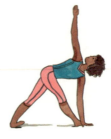

4. Extended Side Angle Pose
30 sec.

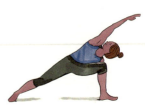

5. Easy Revolved Side Angle Pose
30 sec.

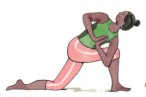

6. Intense Leg Stretch Pose I
30 sec.

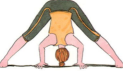

7. Intense Leg Stretch Pose II
30 sec.

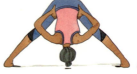

8. Intense Leg Stretch Pose III
30 sec.

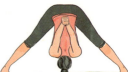

9. Intense Leg Stretch Pose IV
30 sec.

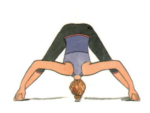

10. Warrior I Pose
30 sec.

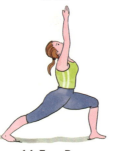

11. Warrior II Pose
30 sec.

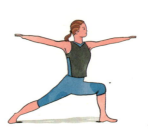

12. Goddess Pose
30-45 sec.

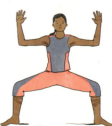

13. Wide-Legged Vinyasa Flow
30-60 sec.

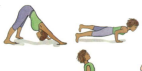

14. Frog Pose
30 sec.

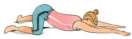

You can support your pelvis with a block or rolled-up towel if needed.

15. Locust Pose
30-60 sec.

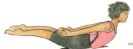

16. Crocodile Pose
30 sec.

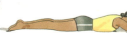

Segment 3: Cool Down

DATE

1. Wide Child's Pose
60 sec.

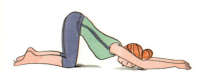

2. Camel Pose w/ Hands to Floor
30 sec.

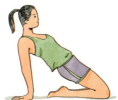

3. Camel Pose
30 sec.

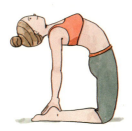

4. Puppy Dog Pose
30-60 sec.

5. Thread the Needle Pose
30 sec. per side

6. Table Top to Child's Pose
30-60 sec.

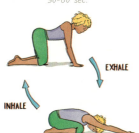

EXHALE
INHALE

7. Staff Pose
30-60 sec.

8. Easy Spinal Twist Pose
30 sec. per side

9. Full-Body Stretch Pose
30 sec.

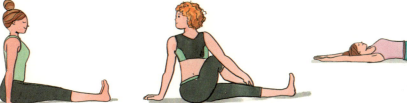

10. Supine Spinal Twist II Pose
30 sec. per side

11. Corpse Pose
5 mins.

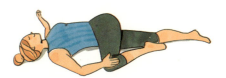
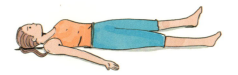

Pro-Tip

Chakras: Sacral Chakra (Svadhisthana).

The second Chakra is located in your pelvic/sacral region just above the Root Chakra. The Sacral Chakra controls the reproductive organs, fosters creativity, and opens us up to be more receptive.

When it's in proper working order, the Sacral Chakra ultimately helps us feel free, flexible, sensual, harmonious, and increased our overall enjoyment in life.

The Sacral Chakra corresponds with these properties:

- **Color** - Orange
- **Element** - Water
- **Sound** - Yam

If your Sacral Chakra is out of whack, that can lead to difficulty expressing and managing emotions, blocked creativity, reproductive issues, and even chronic pain in the lower back and pelvic region.

To return it to a balanced state, focus on asanas that open up the hips and pelvis, such as Goddess Pose, Garland Pose, or Happy Baby Pose.

You can also try soothing your body with a warm bath (essential oils make a great addition to the bath!), doing some creativity exercises, or even just speaking affirmations.

Try something today to help nourish and maintain your Sacral Chakra!

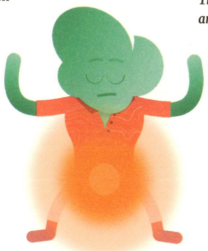

"The yoga pose is not the goal. Becoming flexible is not the goal. Standing on your hands is not the goal. The goal is serenity. Balance. Truly finding peace in your own skin." - Rachel Brathen

Segment 1: Warm-Up

Full Session Exercise Guide:
habitnest.com/pages/yoga-day-25

1. Volcano Pose
60 sec.

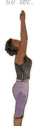

2. Side Lunge
30 sec. per side

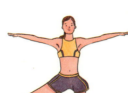

3. Low Lunge w/ Hands to Knee
30 sec. per side

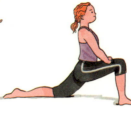

4. Plank to Downward Dog Pose Flow
30-60 sec.

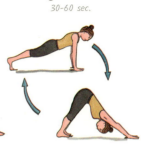

5. Upward-Facing Dog Pose
30 sec.

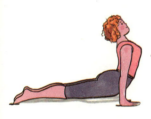

6. Cat-Cow Pose
30-60 sec., alternating

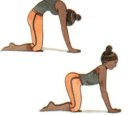

7. Table Top Hip Circles
30-45 sec. each direction

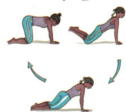

8. Thread the Needle Flow
30 sec. per side

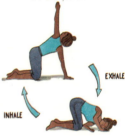

9. Child Pose w/ Arms to One Side
30 sec. per side

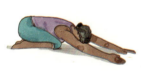

10. Table Top Pose
30 sec.

11. Table Top Pose Wrist Stretch
30 sec.

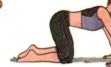

12. Seated Straddle Pose w/ Windshield Wiper Feet
30-60 sec.

13. Upward-Facing Seated Straddle w/ Toe Grab
30-60 sec.

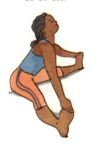

14. Revolved Seated Straddle Pose
30 sec. per side

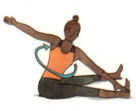

15. Rowing the Boat Flow
30-60 sec.

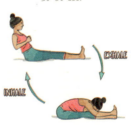

16. Easy Boat Pose w/ Toe Taps
30-60 sec., alternating

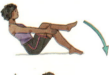
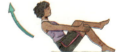

Segment 2: Peak Flow

> Repeat poses 1-4 & 5-8, switching to the opposite side as necessary for asymmetrical poses.

1. Tree Pose
30-60 sec.

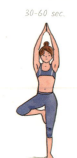

2. Tree Pose w/ Side Bends
30 sec.

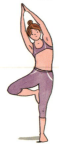

3. Chair Pose
30 sec.

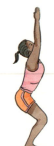

4. Revolved Chair Pose
30 sec.

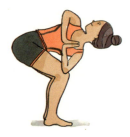

5. Downward Dog to Upward Dog Pose Flow
30 sec.

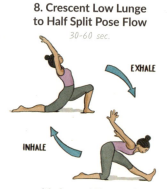

6. Three-Legged Downward-Facing Dog Pose
30 sec.

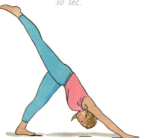

7. Bound Warrior to Humble Warrior Pose Flow
30 sec.

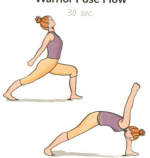

8. Crescent Low Lunge to Half Split Pose Flow
30-60 sec.

9. Crow Pose w/ Toe Taps
30 sec. per side

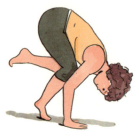

10. Staff Pose
30 sec.

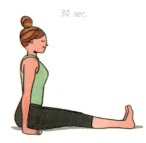

11. Seated Forward Fold Pose
60 sec.

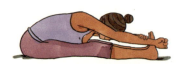

12. Wind Release Pose
60 sec.

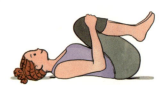

Segment 3: Cool Down

DATE

1. Rolling Happy Baby Variation Flow
60 sec.

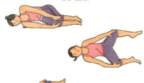

2. Bound Reclined Easy Pose
30-60 sec.

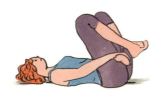

3. Half Plow Pose
30-60 sec.

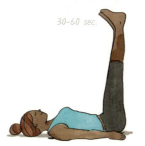

4. Supine Spinal Twist Pose
30 sec. per side

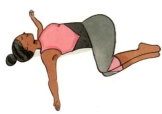

5. Seated Forward Fold Pose
60 sec.

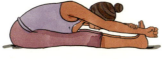

6. Half Happy Baby Pose
30 sec. per side

7. Sitting Swan Pose
30 sec. per side

8. Half Cow Face Pose
30 sec. per side

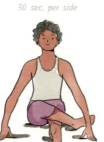

9. Half Cow Face Pose w/ Forward Fold
30 sec. per side

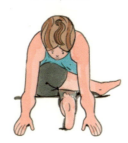

10. Full-Body Stretch Pose
30 sec.

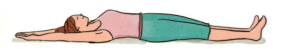

11. Corpse Pose
5 mins.

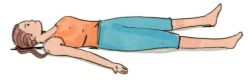

Pro-Tip

Doshas: Pitta.

Moving our way up from the Sacral Chakra, we encounter the Pitta Dosha.

This is the Dosha that's in charge of our metabolism, digestive system, and even our energy levels.

When properly balanced, this Dosha promotes healthy skin, proper digestion, good sleep, and abundant energy.

Those with an imbalance of this Dosha may have a lack of energy, peptic ulcers, heartburn, indigestion, and other issues of the digestive system.

There are tons of ways to promote a balance of the Pitta Dosha in your everyday life, so give it a try!

Here's a few ways you can balance your Pitta Dosha:

- Don't over-schedule yourself
- Eat foods that are sweet or bitter, and foods that are cooling, such as cucumber, melons, or sweet fruits.
- Use candles, incense, or essential oils with sweet, cooling scents like lavender, sandalwood, mint, jasmine, or chamomile
- Spend time in nature
- Balance activity with rest
- Don't skip meals
- Laugh plenty!

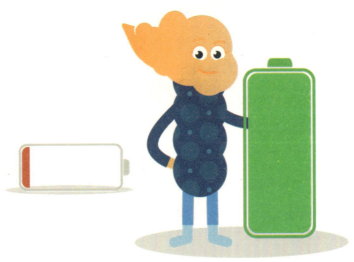

"Yoga is the fountain of youth. You're only as young as your spine is flexible."
- Bob Harper

Segment 1: Warm-Up

Full Session Exercise Guide:
habitnest.com/pages/yoga-day-26

1. Wrist Flexion/ Extension
30 sec.

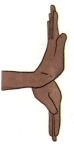

2. Wrist Rotations
30 sec.

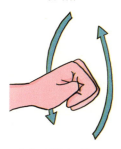

3. Neck Twists
30 sec. each direction

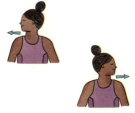

4. Standing Ankle Rotation
30 sec. per side

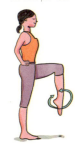

5. Standing Knee Rotation
30 sec. per side

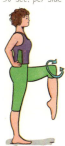

6. Leg Kicks Flow
30 sec. per side

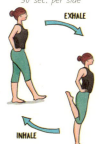

7. Side Lunge Pose w/ Arms Raised
30 sec. per side

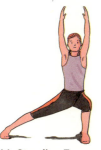

8. Standing Pelvic Circles
30 sec. each direction

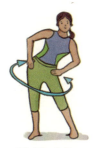

9. Intense Side Stretch
30 sec. per side

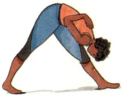

If you can't join your palms, clasp hands behind your back, then extend your arms down.

10. Standing Backbend Pose
60 sec.

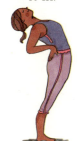

11. Standing Forward Fold Pose
30 sec.

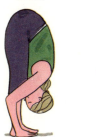

12. Plank Pose w/ Knee-to-Elbow
30 sec. per side

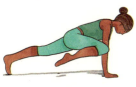

Keep your core engaged and make sure your pelvis/hips don't start dipping or rising up.

13. Forearm Plank Flow
60 sec.

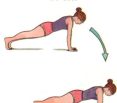

Try to speed it up a little bit each time and see how many reps you can do!

14. Forearm Plank Hip Twists
60 sec., alternating

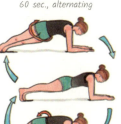

15. Sphinx Pose
60 sec.

16. Sphinx Pose Cat-Cow Flow
30-60 sec.

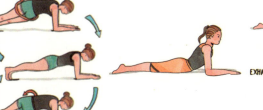
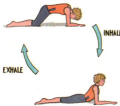

Segment 2: Peak Flow

> Repeat poses 1-12, switching to the opposite side as necessary for asymmetrical poses.

1. Downward Dog to Three-Legged Downward Dog Pose Flow
30-60 sec.

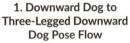

2. Fallen Triangle Pose
30 sec.

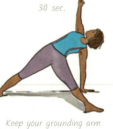

Keep your grounding arm (whichever arm that is supporting you during this pose) stable!

3. Runner's Lunge Pose
30 sec.

4. Triangle Pose Side Stretch
30 sec.

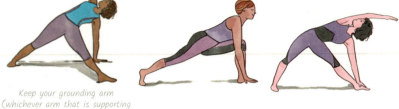

5. Warrior II Pose
30 sec.

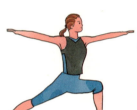

6. Downward Dog to Three-Legged Downward Dog Pose Flow
30 sec.

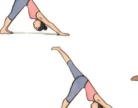

7. Low Lunge Pose
30 sec.

8. Low Lunge w/ Tricep Stretch
30 sec.

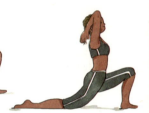

9. High Lunge Pose
30 sec.

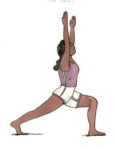

10. Revolved High Lunge Pose
30 sec.

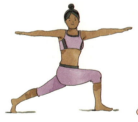

11. Side Lunge Pose
30 sec.

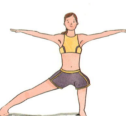

12. Wide-Legged Lateral Squat
30 sec.

13. Plank Pose
30 sec.

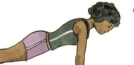

14. Vinyasa II
30-60 sec.

15. Thunderbolt Pose
30-60 sec.

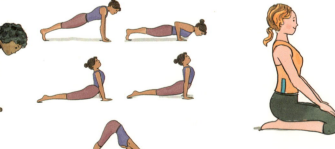

Segment 3: Cool Down

DATE

1. Thunderbolt Pose Salute
30-60 sec.

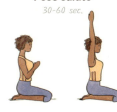

2. Puppy Dog Pose
30-60 sec.

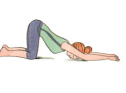

3. Staff Pose
30 sec.

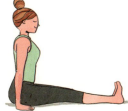

4. Seated Forward Fold Pose
60 sec.

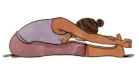

5. Sitting Swan Pose
30 sec. per side

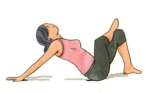

6. Upward-Facing Seated Straddle Pose
30-60 sec.

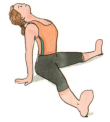

7. Seated Straddle Pose w/ Head-to-Forearms
30-60 sec.

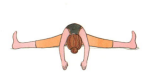

8. Cosmic Egg Pose
30-60 sec.

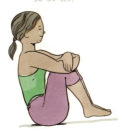

9. Happy Baby Pose
30-60 sec.

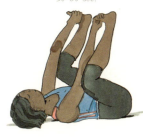

10. Reclining Bound Angle Pose
60 sec.

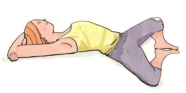

11. Constructive Rest Pose
30-60 sec.

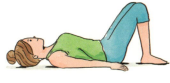

12. Supine Spinal Twist Pose
30 sec. per side

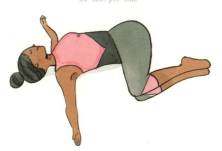

13. Corpse Pose
5 mins.

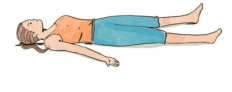

Actionable Challenge

Pranayama: Three-Part Breath

Three-Part Breath, or Dirga Pranayama, is a helpful technique that allows you to prepare for and transition into your flow for the day.

Many teachers begin classes with this breathing exercise to help their students shake off their worries, turn their awareness inward, and tune in to their practice. It's also great for addressing panic attacks, or simply relieving stress throughout the day.

Before starting your flow for the day, take some time to practice this simple breath technique and really attune your mind to your practice.

1. Choose a comfortable spot to sit, or lay supine on your mat. Close your eyes and relax your body completely.

2. Begin by breathing completely naturally, observing the sensations and flow of your breath. If distracting thoughts arise, remember to acknowledge them, and then let the float away as you return your attention to your breathing.

3. For 5 Breaths, breathe through your nose, inhaling deeply with your diaphragm so that your belly rises. As you exhale, draw your belly button inward to expel any remaining air.

4. On your next inhale, breathe deeply and fill your belly with air again. When it's full, inhale just a tiny sip more, expanding into the rib cage. Exhale, releasing air first from the ribcage, then slowly deflating your belly. Repeat for 5 breath cycles.

5. Inhale again, this time expanding your belly, then your rib cage, then all the way up to the collarbone. Exhale, slowly lowering your chest, rib cage, and belly back down. Repeat for 5-10 breath cycles, or until you feel comfortable with it.

Make sure you don't overfill your lungs to the point of feeling uncomfortable or like they're going to burst. Don't strain your breath; allow it to flow in and out, gentle and smooth. If you start to feel dizzy or uncomfortable, return to normal breathing.

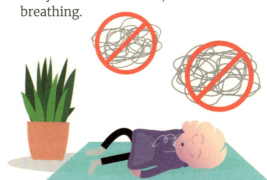

Actionable Challenge Completed:

"What is essential in the practice of yoga is the breath because each pose, each movement, originates from there." - T.K.V. Desikachar

Segment 1: Warm-Up

Full Session Exercise Guide:
habitnest.com/pages/yoga-day-27

1. Three-Part Breath
2 mins.

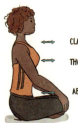

2. Seated Neck Rolls
30 sec. each direction

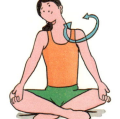

3. Wrist Rolls w/ Hands Clasped
30 sec.

4. Seated Torso Circles
30 sec. each direction

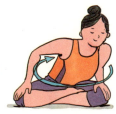

5. Seated Butterfly Pose Wings
60 sec. per side

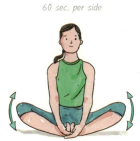

6. Fish Pose w/ Butterfly Legs
60 sec.

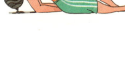

7. Bound Angle Upward Plank Pose Flow
30-60 sec.

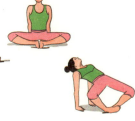

8. Seated Star Pose
60 sec.

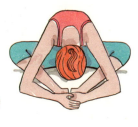

9. Thread the Needle Pose Flow
30 sec. per side

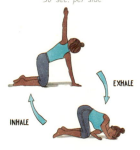

10. Table Top Pose w/ Knee Lift
30 sec.

11. Table Top Pose Lifted Knee Cat-Cow Flow
30 sec.

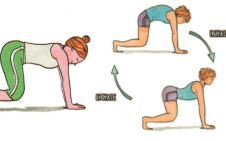

12. Downward-Facing Dog Pose
30-60 sec.

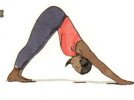

13. Dangling Pose
60 sec.

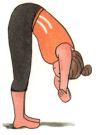

14. Standing Roll-Up Flow
30 sec.

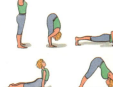

15. Sun Salutation Variation A
~1-2 mins.

16. Sun Salutation Variation B
~1-2 mins.

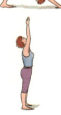
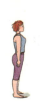

Segment 2: Peak Flow

> Repeat poses 1-12, switching to the opposite side as necessary for asymmetrical poses.

1. Chair Pose
30 sec.

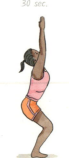

2. Straight-Legged Warrior I Salute Flow
30 sec.

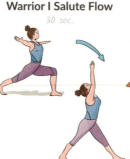

3. Warrior II Intense Leg Stretch Flow
60 sec.

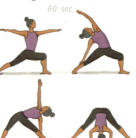

4. Revolved Wide-Legged Forward Fold Pose
30-60 sec.

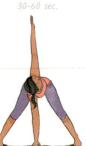

5. Goddess Pose
30-45 sec.

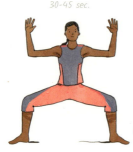

6. Warrior II Pose
30 sec.

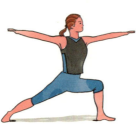

7. Reverse Warrior Pose
30 sec.

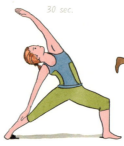

8. Warrior III Pose
30 sec.

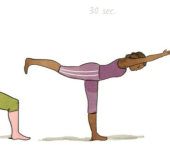

9. Sugarcane Pose
30 sec.

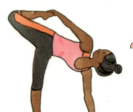

10. Half Moon Pose
30 sec.

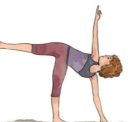

11. Dancer Pose
30 sec.

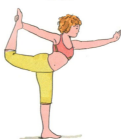

12. Standing Forward Fold Pose
30-60 sec.

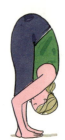

13. Garland Pose
30 sec.

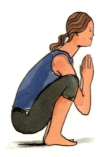

14. Bound Angle Pose
60 sec.

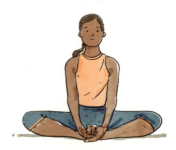

Segment 3: Cool Down

DATE

1. Staff Pose
60 sec.

2. Half Lord of the Fishes Pose
30 sec. per side

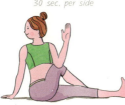

3. Staff Pose w/ Feet Movements
30 sec.

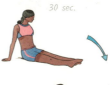

4. Fish Pose Backbend Flow
60 sec.

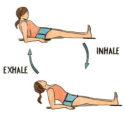

5. Caterpillar Pose
30 sec.

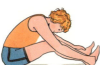

6. Seated Forward Fold Pose
60 sec.

7. Bridge Pose
30-60 sec.

8. Half Wind Release Pose
30 sec. per side

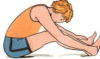

9. Wind Release Pose w/ Knee to Nose
30-60 sec.

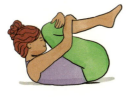

10. Happy Baby Pose
30-60 sec.

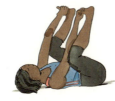

11. Full-Body Stretch Pose
30 sec.

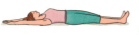

12. Banana Pose
30 sec. per side

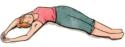

13. Supine Spinal Twist II Pose
30 sec. per side

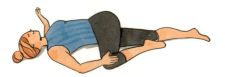

14. Corpse Pose
5 mins.

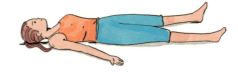

Food for Thought

Koshas: Pranamaya.

The second layer of the Koshas is the Pranamaya Kosha, and it helps to control and regulate our prana, the vital, universal life force comprised of energy that flows in and around us.

While the first layer was about our physical body, this layer is all about the subtle body (the elements of our being that can't be seen or interacted with).

Strengthening this Kosha can help your vital life force flow freely, so it still benefits the health and well-being of your physical body.

The best way to tap into and strengthen your Pranamaya Kosha is through:

- Forming a breath-body connection during your daily yoga flow.
- Performing helpful Pranayama breathing exercises.
- Taking good care of your physical health.

Note: this Kosha is PranaMAYA, and breath control exercises are PranaYAMA.

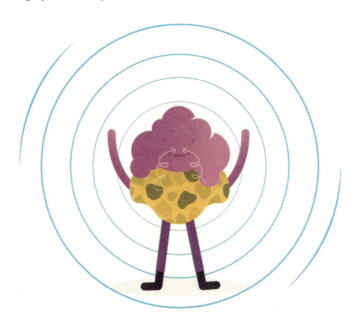

"The body is your temple. Keep it pure and clean for the soul to reside in."
- B.K.S. Iyengar

Segment 1: Warm-Up

Full Session Exercise Guide:
habitnest.com/pages/yoga-day-28

1. Seated Neck Rolls
30 sec. each direction

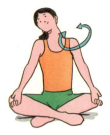

2. Easy Pose Mudra Flow
30 sec.

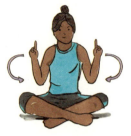

3. Seated Shoulder Rolls
30 sec. forward & backward

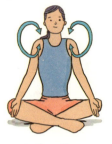

4. Cactus Arms Shoulder Movements
60 sec., alternating

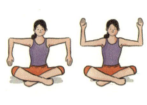

5. Deltoid Stretch
30 sec. per side

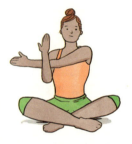

6. Side-to-Side Neck Stretch
30 sec. per side

7. Easy Pose Side Bend
30 sec. per side

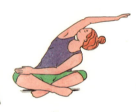

8. Revolved Easy Pose Salute Flow
30-60 sec., alternating

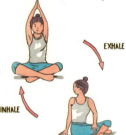

9. Seated Cat-Cow Pose
30-60 sec., alternating

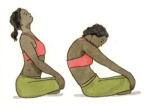

10. Staff Pose
30 sec.

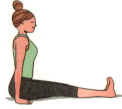

11. Seated Side Straddle Pose
30 sec. per side

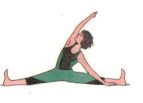

12. Upward-Facing Seated Straddle w/ Toe Grab
30-60 sec.

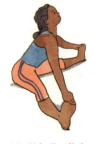

13. Seated Forward Fold Pose
60 sec.

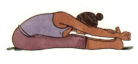

14. Supine Spinal Twist Pose
30 sec. per side

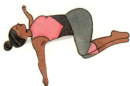

15. Side Reclining Scissors Flow
30-60 sec. per side

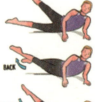

16. Side Reclining Leg Lift
30-60 sec. per side

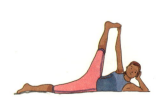

Segment 2: Peak Flow

> Repeat poses 1-8, switching to the opposite side as necessary for asymmetrical poses.

1. Three-Legged Downward-Facing Dog Pose
30 sec.

2. Three-Legged Downward-Facing Dog Pose w/ Knee Rotations
30 sec.

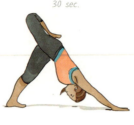

3. Runner's Lunge Pose
30 sec.

4. Warrior I Pose
30 sec.

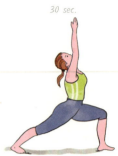

5. Warrior II Pose
30 sec.

6. Reverse Warrior Pose
30 sec.

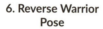

7. Humble Warrior Pose
30 sec.

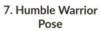

8. Vinyasa I
30 sec.

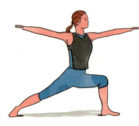
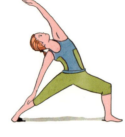
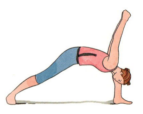

9. Sphinx Pose
30 sec.

10. Locust Pose
30-60 sec.

11. Easy Half Bow Pose
30 sec. per side

12. Bow Pose
30-60 sec.

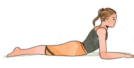
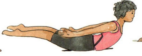
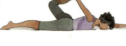
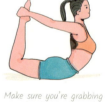

Close your eyes and focus on maintaining slow, steady breaths.

Make sure you're grabbing your feet/ankles from the outside, not the inside.

13. Crocodile Pose
30 sec.

14. Downward Dog Plank Pose Flow
30 sec.

15. Side Plank Pose
30 sec. per side

16. Child's Pose
30-60 sec.

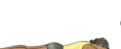
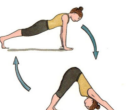
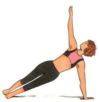
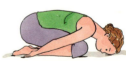

Segment 3: Cool Down

DATE

1. Bound Angle Pose
60 sec.

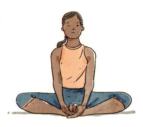

2. Seated Star Pose
60 sec.

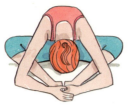

3. Fish Pose w/ Butterfly Legs
60 sec.

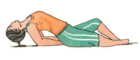

4. Staff Pose
30 sec.

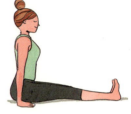

5. Half Lord of the Fishes Pose
30 sec. per side

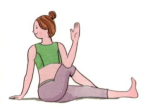

6. Seated Forward Fold Pose
60 sec.

7. Upward-Facing Seated Straddle Pose
30-60 sec.

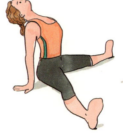

8. Revolved Head-to-Knee Pose
30 sec. per side

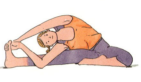

9. Bridge Pose
30-60 sec.

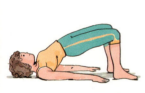

10. Staff Pose w/ Hands Back
15-20 sec.

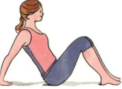

11. Reverse Table Top Pose
30 sec.

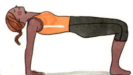

12. Reclined Hand-to-Big-Toe Pose
30 sec. per side

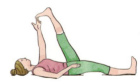

13. Reverse Pigeon Pose
30 sec. per side

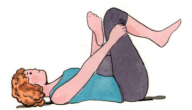

14. Corpse Pose
30-60 sec.

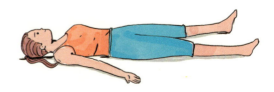

Food for Thought

Yamas: Asteya.

Asteya focuses on more than just the physical act of stealing; it aims to address the greed and insecurity that often fuels the desire to steal from others.

When the desire to steal arises, it's often due to a lack of faith in your ability to achieve and obtain things on your own; a sense that you're not enough, or that you feel you're lacking in some way.

Those feelings tend to spill over into other areas of life, taking your focus away from your inner journey. It leads to unhealthy comparisons between yourself and others, pushing yourself too hard, and negative self-talk.

An imbalance in this Yama can also lead to hoarding unnecessary items and stressful clutter.

Here's how you can practice it in everyday life:

- De-clutter and organize your work and living spaces.
- Foster self-care and acceptance to combat the sense of lacking or low self-worth.
- During your practice, focus on how the poses feel, not how you think they should look.
- Don't push yourself past what feels right for you.
- Use affirmations such as "I am enough".

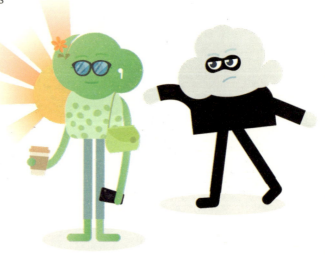

"It's not about being good at something. It's about being good to yourself."
- Unknown

Segment 1: Warm-Up

Full Session Exercise Guide:
habitnest.com/pages/yoga-day-29

1. Corpse Pose
60 sec.

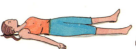

2. Banana Pose
30 sec. per side

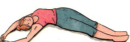

3. Wind Release Pose
60 sec.

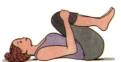

4. Circle of Joy
60 sec.

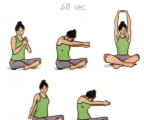

5. Cat-Cow Pose
30-60 sec., alternating

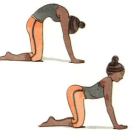

6. Tiger Pose
30 sec. per side

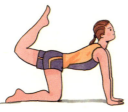

7. Child's Pose w/ Arms to One Side
30 sec. per side

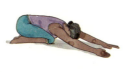

8. Kneeling Sun Salutation
~2 mins.

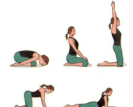

9. Thunderbolt Pose w/ Swinging Arms
30 sec.

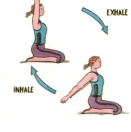

10. Shoulder Socket Rotations
30-60 sec.

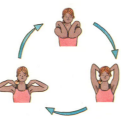

11. Cow Face Arms
30 sec. per side

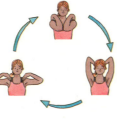

12. Standing Forward Fold Pose
30 sec.

13. Standing Roll-Up Flow
30-60 sec.

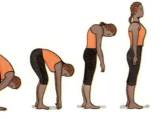

14. Standing Circle of Joy
60 sec.

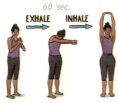

15. Breath of Joy
60-90 sec.

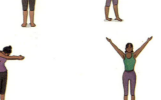
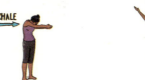

Segment 2: Peak Flow

> Repeat poses 9-16, switching to the opposite side as necessary for asymmetrical poses.

1. Standing Bound Rising Locust Pose
30-60 sec.

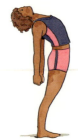

2. Forward Fold Flow
30 sec.

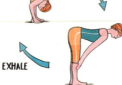

3. Plank Pose
30 sec.

4. Cobra Pose
30-60 sec.

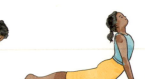

5. Cobra Pose w/ Bow Legs
30 sec.

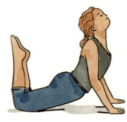

6. Cobra Pose w/ Hands Lifted
30 sec.

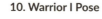

7. Plank to Child's Pose Flow
30 sec.

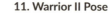

8. Child's Pose Sphinx Flow
30-60 sec.

9. Downward Dog to Three-Legged Downward Dog Flow
30 sec.

10. Warrior I Pose
30 sec.

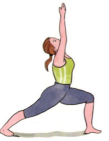

11. Warrior II Pose
30 sec.

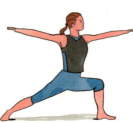

12. Triangle Pose
30 sec.

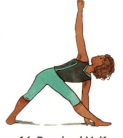

13. Crescent Low Lunge Pose
30 sec.

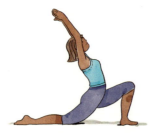

14. Twisted Low Lunge Pose
30 sec.

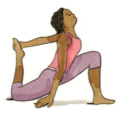

15. Half Splits Pose
30-60 sec.

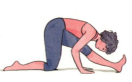

16. Revolved Half Splits Pose
30 sec.

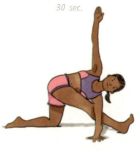

Segment 3: Cool Down

DATE

1. Thunderbolt Pose w/ Cat-Cow
30 sec.

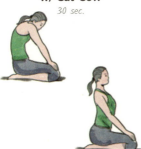

2. Revolved Thunderbolt Pose
30 sec. per side

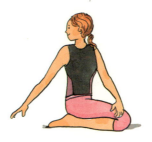

3. Thunderbolt Pose Salute
60 sec.

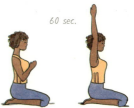
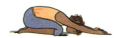

4. Puppy Dog Pose
30-60 sec.

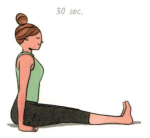

5. Resting Half Frog Pose
30 sec. per side

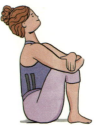

6. Seated Wind Release Pose
30-60 sec.

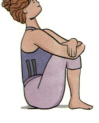

7. Staff Pose
30 sec.

8. Seated Forward Fold Pose
60 sec.

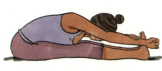
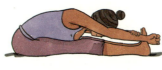

9. Sitting Swan Pose
30 sec. per side

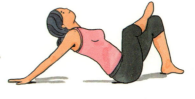

10. Happy Baby Pose
30-60 sec.

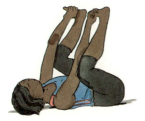

11. Reclining Bound Angle Pose
30-60 sec.

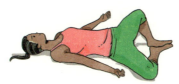

12. Corpse Pose
5 mins.

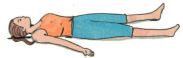

Food for Thought

Niyamas: Tapas (self-discipline).

Tapas translates to 'austerity' or 'discipline', with the Sanskrit root word 'tap' meaning 'to burn.'

It encourages a burning passion, commitment, and desire for growth.

It instills courage in the face of obstacles, and it promotes consistency.

Note that this **does not** mean pushing yourself to the extreme.

It's about sticking to your practice, habits, and routines, and continuing to pursue growth on and off the mat.

Here are a few ways you can cultivate Tapas in life & in your yoga practice:

- Show up for your yoga routine, even if it's only for a short time.
- Keep your promises and do what you say you're going to do.
- Keep your actions aligned with your goals and core values.
- Replace negative inner thoughts with positive affirmations.
- Do exercises that focus on core strength.
- Don't give up!

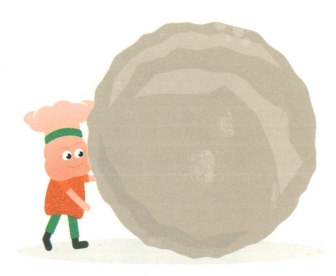

"True success is achieved by stretching oneself, learning to feel comfortable being uncomfortable." - Ken Poirot

Segment 1: Warm-Up

Full Session Exercise Guide:
habitnest.com/pages/yoga-day-30

1. Bound Angle Pose
60 sec.

2. Cradle Pose
30 sec. per side

3. Head-to-Knee Pose
30 sec. per side

4. Revolved Head-to-Knee Pose
30 sec. per side

5. Crocodile Pose
30 sec.

6. Locust Pose
30-60 sec.

7. Dolphin Pose
60 sec.

8. Three-Legged Downward-Facing Dog Pose
30 sec. per side

9. Lizard Pose
30-60 sec. per side

10. Triangle Pose w/ Bent Knee
30 sec. per side

11. Standing Forward Fold Pose
30 sec.

12. Dangling Pose
30-60 sec.

13. Chair Pose
30 sec.

14. Standing Backbend Pose
30-60 sec.

> Repeat poses 8-10, switching to the opposite side as necessary for asymmetrical poses.

Segment 2: Peak Flow

> Repeat poses 1-12, switching to the opposite side as necessary for asymmetrical poses.

1. Chair Pose
30 sec.

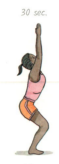

2. Straight-Legged Warrior I Salute Flow
30 sec.

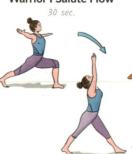

3. Warrior II Intense Leg Stretch Flow
60 sec.

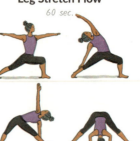

4. Revolved Wide-Legged Forward Fold Pose
30-60 sec.

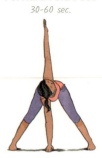

5. Goddess Pose
30-45 sec.

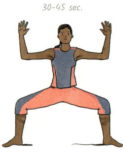

6. Warrior II Pose
30 sec.

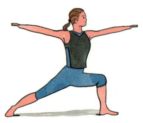

7. Reverse Warrior Pose
30 sec.

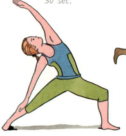

8. Warrior III Pose
30 sec.

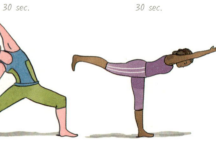

9. Sugarcane Pose
30 sec.

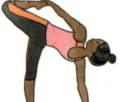

10. Half Moon Pose
30 sec.

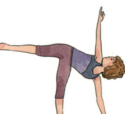

11. Dancer Pose
30 sec.

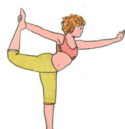

12. Standing Forward Fold Pose
30-60 sec.

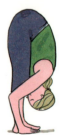

13. Garland Pose
30 sec.

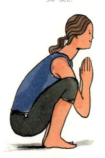

14. Bound Angle Pose
60 sec.

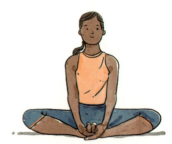

Segment 3: Cool Down

DATE

1. Rolling Happy Baby Variation Flow
60 sec.

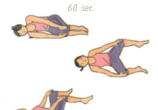

2. Bound Reclined Easy Pose
30-60 sec.

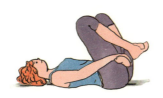

3. Half Plow Pose
30-60 sec.

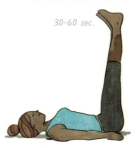

4. Supine Spinal Twist Pose
30 sec. per side

5. Seated Forward Fold Pose
60 sec.

6. Half Happy Baby Pose
30 sec. per side

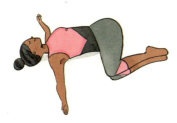
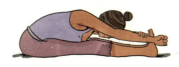

7. Sitting Swan Pose
30 sec. per side

8. Half Cow Face Pose
30 sec. per side

9. Half Cow Face Pose w/ Forward Fold
30 sec. per side

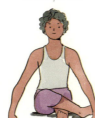
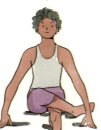
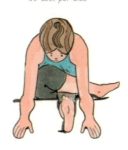

10. Full-Body Stretch Pose
30 sec.

11. Corpse Pose
5 mins.

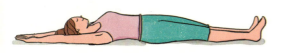
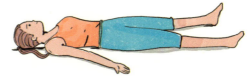

Actionable Challenge

Pranayama: inhale the nectar.

Using visualization and engaging your senses can be a great way of deepening your practice and creating more mindfulness.

This exercise is an easy way to connect with your breath and soothe your body, and it can be done virtually anywhere, so give it a shot!

Try this super quick trick:

1. Close your eyes, open your mouth, and inhale deeply with your diaphragm.

2. As you inhale, imagine that the air tastes like sweet nectar. Taste the air, imagining the sweetness, visualizing that this nectar contains the love and support of the universe, and it's flowing into you.

3. Watch as your belly and lower rib cage expand, truly absorbing that life-sustaining love and support from the universe.

4. Hold it for a short count, then exhale, imagining that everything good that was in the air remains even as the breath recedes.

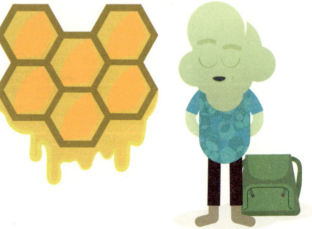

"Yoga does not just change the way we see things, it transforms the person who sees." - B.K.S. Iyengar

Segment 1: Warm-Up

Full Session Exercise Guide:
habitnest.com/pages/yoga-day-31

1. Reclining Bound Angle Pose
60 sec.

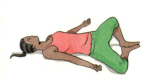

2. Revolved Abdomen Twist Pose
60 sec.

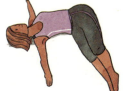

3. Forward-to-Backward Neck Stretch
30-60 sec., alternating

4. Side-to-Side Neck Stretches
30 sec. per side

5. Alternating Shoulder Shrugs
30 sec.

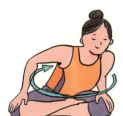

6. Seated Torso Circles
30 sec. each direction

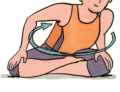

7. Seated Forward Fold Prep
60 sec.

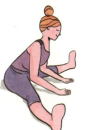

8. Seated Straddle Prep
30-60 sec.

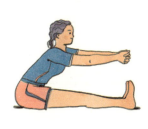

9. Sage Marichi Pose C
30 sec. per side

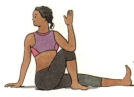

10. Seated Forward Fold Pose
60 sec.

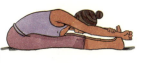

11. Upward Facing Seated Straddle w/ Toe Grab
30-60 sec.

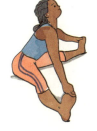

12. Cat-Cow Pose
30-60 sec., alternating

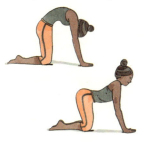

13. Table Top Side-to-Side Flow
30-60 sec.

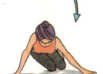

14. Balancing Table Top Knee-to-Nose Flow
30 sec. per side

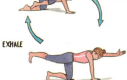

15. Unilateral Balancing Table Top Pose
30 sec. per side

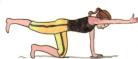

16. Wide Child's Pose
30-60 sec.

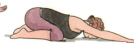

Segment 2: Peak Flow

> Repeat poses 1-8, switching to the opposite side as necessary for asymmetrical poses.

1. Three-Legged Downward Dog to Tiger Pose
30 sec.

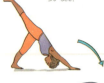

2. Warrior I Pose
30 sec.

3. Revolved Side Angle Pose
30 sec.

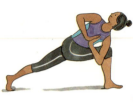

4. Warrior II Pose
30 sec.

5. Standing Archer Pose
30 sec.

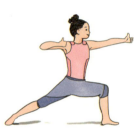

6. Dancing Warrior Pose
30-60 sec.

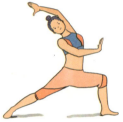

7. Sky Archer Pose
30 sec.

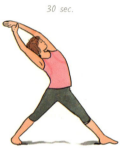

8. Dancer Pose
30 sec.

9. Goddess Pose
30-45 sec.

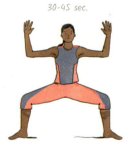

10. Intense Leg Stretch Pose
60 sec.

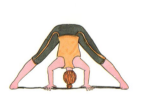

11. Extended Mountain Pose Backbend
30 sec.

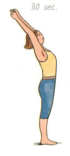

12. Dangling Pose
30-60 sec.

13. Garland Pose
30 sec.

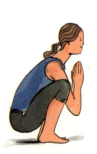

14. Revolved Squat Pose
30 sec. per side

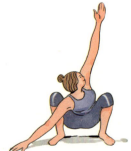

15. Seated Butterfly Pose Wing
30 sec.

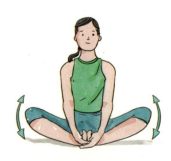

Segment 3: Cool Down

DATE

1. Easy Pose w/ Elbows on Floor
30-60 sec.

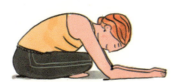

2. Seated Straddle Forward Fold
30-60 sec.

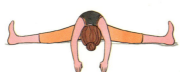

3. Sitting Swan Pose
30 sec. per side

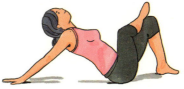

4. Seated Wind Release Pose
30-60 sec.

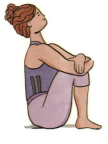

5. Easy Boat Pose
30-60 sec.

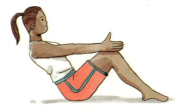

6. Boat Pose B
30 sec.

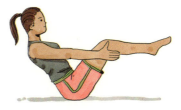

7. Full-Body Stretch Pose
30 sec.

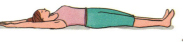

8. Fish Pose
60 sec.

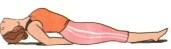

9. Bridge Pose
30-60 sec.

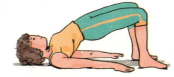

10. Supine Spinal Twist II Pose
30 sec. per side

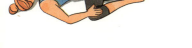

11. Wind Release Pose Breath Flow
30-60 sec.

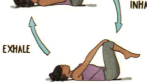

12. Corpse Pose
5 mins.

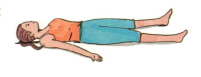

Pro-Tip

Asanas: Mudras & how to use them.

Mudras are another common element found in yoga practices. Mudras are simply hand gestures that are believed to hold deep meaning, redirect and align our energy flow, and help us reach a state of equilibrium.

They essentially manipulate the flow of energy to achieve bodily healing and harmony. They can be performed practically anywhere, and for any length of time.

Before performing Mudras, rub your hands and get your circulation flowing first! Your hands need to warm up and prepare, just like the rest of the body.

Common Mudras:

- **Anjali Mudra** — otherwise known as 'prayer hands' or 'namaste hands', this Mudra is performed by joining the palms of your hands in front of your chest.

- **Gyana Mudra** — also called the 'Mudra of Knowledge', this Mudra is done by placing your hands palm-up on your lap, joining the tip of the index finger to the thumb, and stretching the other 3 fingers out straight.

- **Vayu Mudra** — this Mudra is said to reduce pain and discomfort, stimulate your immune system, and regulate your digestive system. Simply place both hands on your lap with palms up, fold your index finger down, then gently hold it down by placing your thumb near your 2nd knuckle. Keep the remaining fingers outstretched.

- **Prana Mudra** — this life-force boosting Mudra is done by touching the tip of the ring and middle finger to the tip of your thumb, keeping the other 2 fingers outstretched.

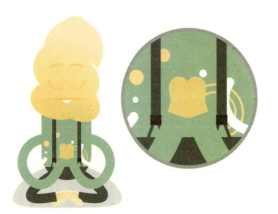

"The word mudra literally means "a seal." Mudras are a subtle science of arranging your body in a certain way." - Sadhguru

Segment 1: Warm-Up

Full Session Exercise Guide:
habitnest.com/pages/yoga-day-32

1. Seated Neck Rolls
30 sec. each direction

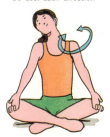

2. Seated Torso Circles
30 sec. each direction

3. Cosmic Egg Pose
60 sec.

4. Seated Cat-Cow Pose
30-60 sec., alternating

5. Mountain Pose Arm Warm-Up
60 sec.

6. Palm Tree Pose
30-60 sec.

7. Palm Tree Pose w/ Side Bend
30 sec. per side

8. Standing Bound Rising Locust Pose
60 sec.

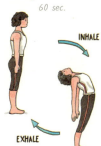

9. Standing Pelvic Circles
30 sec. each direction

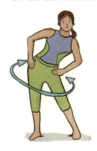

10. Standing Quad Stretch
30 sec. per side

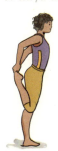

11. Squat w/ Arms Crossed
30-60 sec.

12. Side Lunge Pose
30 sec. per side

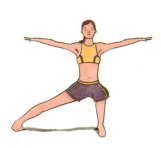

13. Chair Pose
30 sec.

14. Half Forward Fold Pose
30-60 sec.

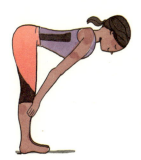

Segment 2: Peak Flow

Repeat poses 1-4 & 5-8, switching to the opposite side as necessary for asymmetrical poses.

1. Tree Pose
30-60 sec.

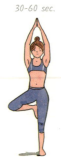

2. Tree Pose w/ Side Bends
30 sec.

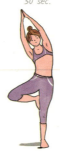

3. Chair Pose
30 sec.

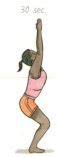

4. Revolved Chair Pose
30 sec.

5. Downward Dog to Upward Dog Pose Flow
30 sec.

6. Three-Legged Downward-Facing Dog Pose
30 sec.

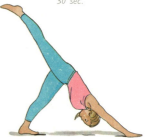

7. Bound Warrior to Humble Warrior Pose Flow
30-60 sec.

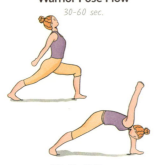

8. Crescent Low Lunge to Half Split Pose Flow
30-60 sec.

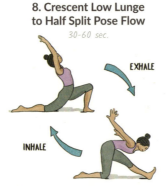

9. Crow Pose w/ Toe Taps
30 sec. per side

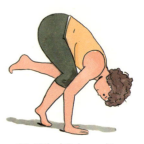

10. Staff Pose
30 sec.

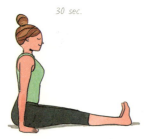

11. Seated Forward Fold Pose
60 sec.

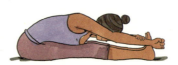

12. Wind Release Pose
60 sec.

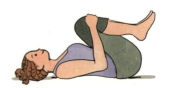

Segment 3: Cool Down

DATE

1. Reclining Bound Angle Pose
60 sec.

2. Supine Butterfly Wings Flow
30-60 sec.

3. Banana Pose w/ Ankles Crossed
30 sec. per side

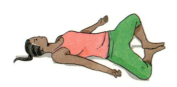
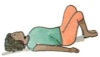
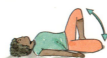
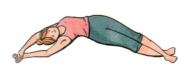

4. Wind Release Pose
60 sec.

5. Supine Spinal Twist II Pose
30 sec. per side

6. Happy Baby Pose
30-60 sec.

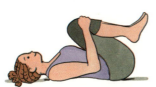
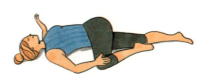
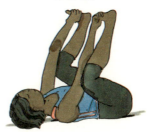

7. Reclined Cow Face Pose
30 sec., then reverse legs & repeat

8. Cat Pulling Tail Pose
30 sec. per side

9. Supine Spinal Twist Shoulder Stretch Flow
30 sec. per side

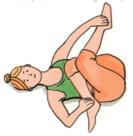
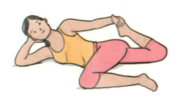
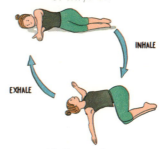

10. Crocodile Pose
30 sec.

11. Easy Half Bow Pose
30 sec. per side

12. Corpse Pose
5 mins.

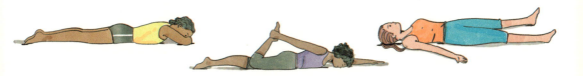

Actionable Challenge

Pratyahara: do your yoga completely distraction-free.

To achieve a deep meditative state, it's essential that you reduce distractions as much as possible.

When you perform your next yoga routine, challenge yourself to have a truly distraction-free flow.

If you're not sure what steps to take to eliminate distractions, here are some options:

- *Put your phone on silent and stash it somewhere out of sight.* Phones and other unnecessary devices are a common obstacle for the modern Yogi. All it takes is one notification to pull us away from our focus and get us sucked back into the screen.

- *Make sure the room is set to a comfortable temperature.* It's hard to stay focused when you feel like you're going to pass out from the heat or you're shivering from the cold.

- *Make sure your yoga space is clean and de-cluttered.* Clutter and mess are enemies of focus!

- *Keep any props you might need during your flow nearby* so that you can easily grab them without stepping away from the mat.

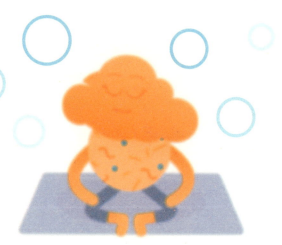

Actionable Challenge Completed: ☐

"Through sustained focus and meditation on our patterns, habits, and conditioning, we gain knowledge and understanding of our past and how we can change the patterns that aren't serving us to live more freely and fully." - Patañjali

Segment 1: Warm-Up

Full Session Exercise Guide:
habitnest.com/pages/yoga-day-33

1. Easy Pose
30-60 sec.

2. Easy Pose Warm-Up
1-2 mins.

3. Cat-Cow to Child's Pose Flow
1-2 mins.

4. Thread the Needle Flow
30 sec. per side

5. Table Top Pose w/ Leg Raise
30 sec. per side

6. Supported Side Plank
30 sec. per side

7. Low Lunge w/ Hands to Knee
30 sec. per side

8. One-Legged Bow Pose
30 sec. per side

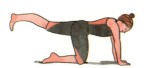
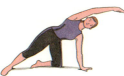
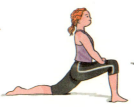
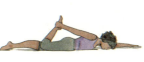

9. Vinyasa I
30 sec.

10. Mountain Pose
30 sec.

11. Standing Wind Release Pose
30 sec. per side

12. Mountain Pose w/ Twist
30 sec. per side

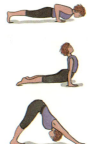
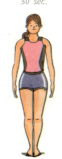
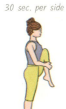

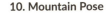
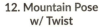

13. Standing Backbend Pose
30-60 sec.

14. Standing Forward Fold w/ Knees Bent
30-60 sec.

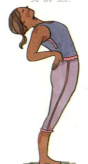
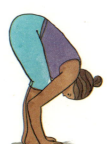
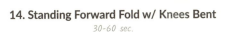
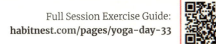

Segment 2: Peak Flow

> Repeat poses 5-8 & 9-12, switching to the opposite side as necessary for asymmetrical poses.

1. Tree Pose
30-60 sec.

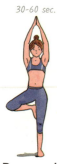

2. Upward Salute Side Bend
30 sec. each side

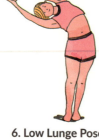

3. Chair Pose
30 sec.

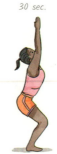

4. Forward Fold Flow
30 sec.

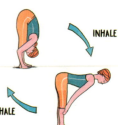

5. Downward Dog Crescent Lunge Flow
60 sec.

6. Low Lunge Pose w/ Cat-Cow
30 sec.

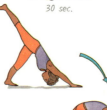

Don't use your hands to push or pull your neck/head at all. Simply rest your hands there.

7. Crescent Low Lunge to Revolved Side Angle Pose Flow
30-60 sec.

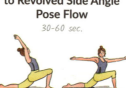

8. Vinyasa I
30 sec.

9. Downward Dog to Plank Pose Flow
30 sec.

10. Three-Legged Downward Dog to Tiger Pose
30 sec.

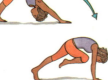

11. Pigeon Pose
30 sec.

12. One-Legged King Pigeon Prep
30 sec.

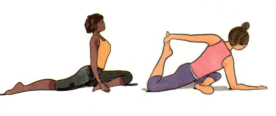

13. Reverse Corpse Pose
30 sec.

14. Prone to Supine Corpse Pose Flow
30-60 sec.

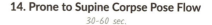
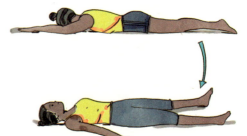
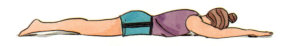

Segment 3: Cool Down

DATE

1. Wind Release Pose
60 sec.

2. Happy Baby Pose
30-60 sec.

3. Supine Spinal Twist II Pose
30 sec. per side

4. Staff Pose
30 sec.

5. Sage Marichi C Pose
30 sec. per side

6. Upward-Facing Seated Straddle Pose
30-60 sec.

7. Seated Straddle Pose
30-60 sec.

8. Head-to-Knee Pose
30 sec. per side

9. Seated Forward Fold Pose
60 sec.

10. Easy Pose
30-60 sec.

11. Reclining Bound Angle Pose
30-60 sec.

12. Corpse Pose
5 mins.

Actionable Challenge

Dharana: Set an intention for your flow of the day.

Before you begin your daily yoga flow, take the time to set a Sankalpa (intention).

Setting an intention brings more mindfulness and thoughtful action to your yoga practice and your life.

Intentions are meant to be positive and provide value, and they focus on what you can/will do rather than what you can't/won't do.

For example, instead of choosing *"I won't judge myself or others"* as an intention, try *"I am a non-judgmental safe space for myself and others."*

Intentions direct your focus toward some sort of quality or virtue that you want to work toward or cultivate more of in your life.

An intention can be anything that brings joy, happiness, and overall well-being.

For example:
- "I am kind and compassionate."
- "I show myself love and acceptance."
- "I will cultivate more balance in my life."
- "My heart and mind are open and receptive."

Try setting one today! Start by closing your eyes and tuning into your breath, then choose an intention to dedicate the day's practice to.

Don't just say a string of words that you think you're *supposed* to say; make your intention heartfelt and genuine.

Revisit your intention later if you feel yourself falling off track or losing focus!

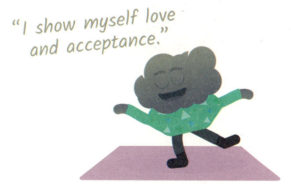

"I show myself love and acceptance."

Actionable Challenge Completed: ☐

"It is indeed true that by practicing yoga we gradually improve our ability to concentrate and be independent. We improve our health, our relationships, and everything we do." - T.K.V. Desikachar

Segment 1: Warm-Up

Full Session Exercise Guide:
habitnest.com/pages/yoga-day-34

1. Constructive Rest Pose w/ Arms Overhead

30-60 sec.

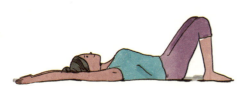

2. Cycling Pose

60-90 sec., alternating legs

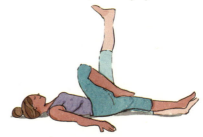

3. Supine Windshield Wipers

30 sec. per side

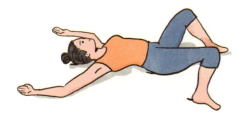

4. Reclined Half Cow Face Pose

30-60 sec. per side

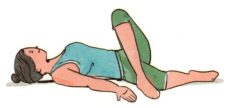

5. Reclined Hand-to-Big-Toe Pose

30 sec. per side

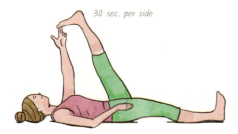

6. Reverse Pigeon Pose

30 sec. per side

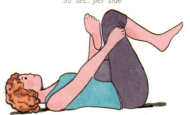

7. Supine Spinal Twist II Pose

30 sec. per side

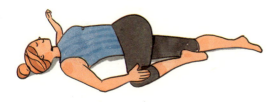

8. Reclined Cow Face Pose

30 sec., then reverse legs & repeat

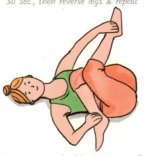

Make sure your shoulder blades stay flat on the floor, pulled away from each other.

Segment 2: Peak Flow

> Repeat poses 1-7 & 9-12, switching to the opposite side as necessary for asymmetrical poses.

1. Downward-Facing Dog Pose
30 sec.

2. Downward Dog Plank Flow
30 sec.

3. Forward Fold Flow
30 sec.

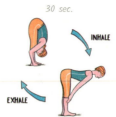

4. Volcano Pose
30 sec.

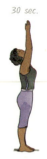

5. Tree Pose
30 sec.

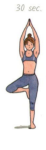

6. Dancer Pose
30 sec.

7. Warrior I Pose
30 sec.

8. Downward Dog to Mountain Pose Flow
30-45 sec.

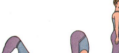

9. Downward-Facing Dog Pose
30 sec.

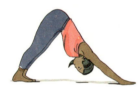

10. Plank Pose
30 sec.

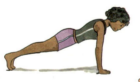

11. Side Plank Pose
30 sec.

12. Wild Thing Pose
30 sec.

13. Wide Child's Pose
30 sec.

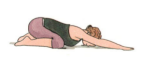

14. Eight-Limbed Striking Cobra Flow
30 sec.

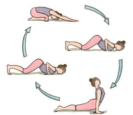

15. Puppy Dog Pose
30-60 sec.

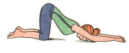

16. Child's Pose
30-60 sec.

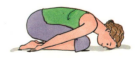

Segment 3: Cool Down

DATE

1. Thread the Needle Pose
30 sec. per side

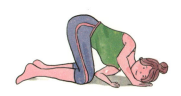

2. Striking Cobra Pose
60 sec.

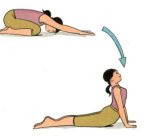

3. Easy Half Bow Pose
30 sec. per side

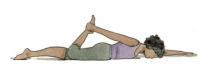

4. Half Wind Release Pose
30 sec. per side

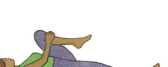

5. Happy Baby Pose
30-60 sec.

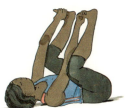

6. Supine Abdominal Twist
30 sec. per side

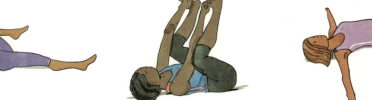

7. Staff Pose
30 sec.

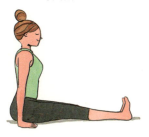

8. Bharadvaja's Twist Pose
30 sec. per side

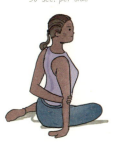

9. Easy Boat Pose
30-60 sec.

10. Upward Plank Pose
30-60 sec.

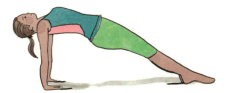

11. Corpse Pose
5 mins.

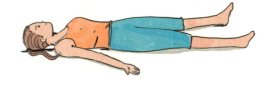

Actionable Challenge

Dhyana: body scan meditation.

Body scan meditations are very similar to the meditative process we use during Savasana. In fact, you can use body scan meditation during Savasana to enhance your experience and mindfulness.

This form of meditation also allows you to tune in to your body, noticing all of the sensations and relaxing your body more deeply than ever. It also teaches us to address the unpleasant things in life, sit with them, and move on from them.

During your next Savasana, try out this body scan meditation:

1. Get settled comfortably in Corpse Pose (Savasana). Close your eyes and take a moment to tap into your body-breath connection.

2. Start at your toes. Notice the sensations in them and take note of any tightness. In your mind or aloud, say, "I am relaxing my toes. My toes are relaxed now" as you release any tension from them.

3. Repeat this, moving up to your feet, ankles, calves, thighs, and so on, until you've completely relaxed your whole body.

Stay curious about what you're feeling and experiencing, and if your attention begins to wander, gently redirect it back to the meditation!

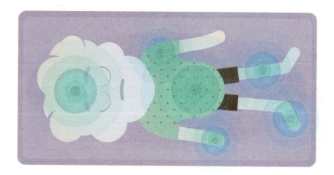

Actionable Challenge Completed: ☐

"Yoga does not always cure stress. It neutralizes it through increasing awareness and by changing self-perception." - Debasish Mridha

Segment 1: Warm-Up

Full Session Exercise Guide:
habitnest.com/pages/yoga-day-35

1. Thunderbolt Pose
30-60 sec.

2. Revolved Thunderbolt Pose
30 sec. per side

3. Kneeling Side Bends
30 sec. per side

4. Cat-Cow Pose
30-60 sec., alternating

5. Child's Pose Sphinx Flow
30-60 sec.

6. Wide Child's Pose
30-60 sec.

7. Wide-Legged Vinyasa Flow
30-60 sec.

8. Downward Dog to Mountain Pose Flow
30 sec.

9. Mountain Pose Tiptoes Flow
30 sec.

10. Standing Arm Circles
30 sec. each direction

11. Easy Joint Warm-Up Flow
1-2 mins.

12. Mountain Pose Forward Fold Arm Swings
30 sec.

13. Standing Wind Release Pose
30 sec. per side

14. Standing Quad Stretch
30 sec. per side

15. Mountain Pose Namaste
30 sec.

Segment 2: Peak Flow

> Repeat poses 1-12, switching to the opposite side as necessary for asymmetrical poses.

1. Five-Pointed Star Pose
30 sec.

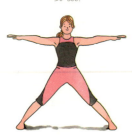

2. Triangle Pose
30 sec.

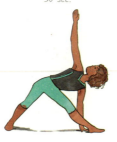

3. Revolved Triangle Pose
30 sec.

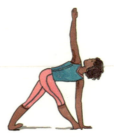

4. Extended Side Angle Pose
30 sec.

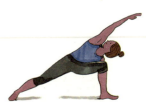

5. Easy Revolved Side Angle Pose
30 sec.

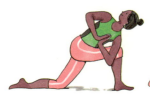

6. Intense Leg Stretch Pose I
30 sec.

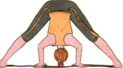

7. Intense Leg Stretch Pose II
30 sec.

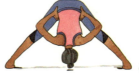

8. Intense Leg Stretch Pose III
30 sec.

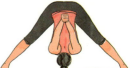

9. Intense Leg Stretch Pose IV
30 sec.

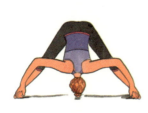

10. Warrior I Pose
30 sec.

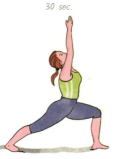

11. Warrior II Pose
30 sec.

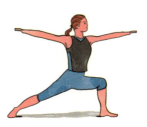

12. Goddess Pose
30-45 sec.

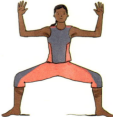

13. Wide-Legged Vinyasa Flow
30-60 sec.

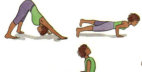

14. Frog Pose
30 sec.

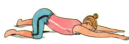

15. Locust Pose
30-60 sec.

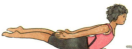

16. Crocodile Pose
30 sec.

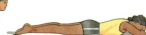

Segment 3: Cool Down

DATE

1. Camel Pose w/ Hands to Floor
30 sec.

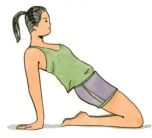

2. Puppy Dog Pose
30-60 sec.

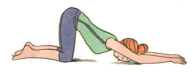

3. Reclined Hero Pose
60 sec.

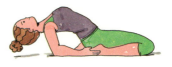

4. Child's Pose
30-60 sec.

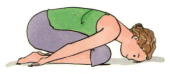

5. Table Top Pose
60 sec.

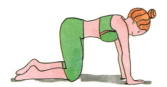

6. Crocodile Pose
30 sec.

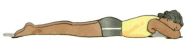

7. Sphinx Pose
60 sec.

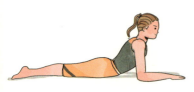

8. Reclining Bound Angle Pose
60 sec.

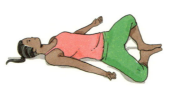

9. Happy Baby Pose
30-60 sec.

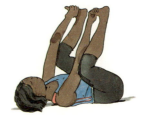

10. Half Wind Release Pose
30 sec. per side

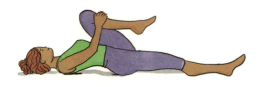

11. Corpse Pose
5 mins.

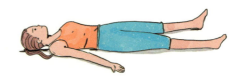

Food for Thought

Chakras: Solar Plexus (Manipura).

The Solar Plexus (or Navel) Chakra is the energy control center located near your belly button that governs digestion, confidence, courage, and sense of inner power.

When properly balanced, this Chakra keeps you feeling supercharged, productive, and motivated!

This Chakra's matching characteristics are:

- **Color** - Yellow
- **Element** - Fire
- **Sound** - Ram

Of course, when this Chakra is blocked or out of balance, you're likely to experience low self-esteem, fatigue, fear, incapability, or stagnancy.

You lose your driving sense of purpose, power, and motivation, so your productivity takes a nosedive. Your digestive system gets disrupted, leading to stomach pain, indigestion, IBS, and other problems.

You can balance this Chakra by:

- Repeating positive, motivational affirmations.
- Performing asanas that balance this Chakra, such as Boat Pose, the Warrior Poses or Sun Salutations.
- Aromatherapy using incense or essential oils like ginger, cinnamon, or sandalwood.
- Heal from past trauma and grief, even if that means seeking counselling.

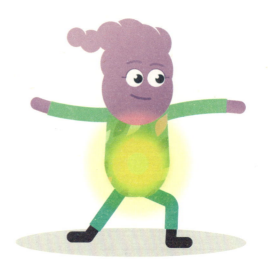

"When we push for immediate results and instant healing, we never inhabit the important in-between phase, which is where much of the learning and growth actually happen." - Bo Forbes

Segment 1: Warm-Up

Full Session Exercise Guide:
habitnest.com/pages/yoga-day-36

1. Toe Flexion/Extension
30 sec.

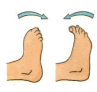

2. Ankle Rotations
30 sec.

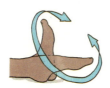

3. Seated Knee Rotations
30 sec. per side

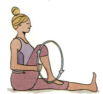

4. Cradle Pose
30 sec. per side

5. Seated Hip Rotations
30 sec. per side

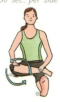

6. Seated Butterfly Wings
30-60 sec.

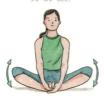

7. Finger Abduction/Adduction
30 sec.

8. Wrist Flexion/Extension
30 sec.

9. Wrist Rotations
30 sec.

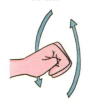

10. Elbow Flexion/Extension
30 sec.

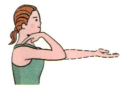

11. Shoulder Socket Rotations
30-60 sec.

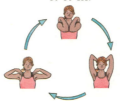

12. Seated Neck Rolls
30 sec. each direction

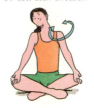

13. Easy Pose Upward Salute
30-60 sec.

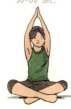

14. Easy Pose Side Bends w/ Fingers Interlocked
30 sec. per side

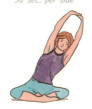

15. Revolved Easy Pose
30 sec. per side

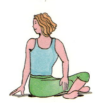

16. Cat-Cow Pose
30-60 sec., alternating

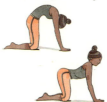

Segment 2: Peak Flow

> Repeat poses 1-8, switching to the opposite side as necessary for asymmetrical poses.

1. Standing Wind Release Pose
30 sec. per side

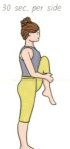

2. Tree Pose
30 sec.

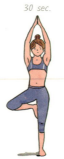

3. Revolved Hand-to-Big-Toe Pose
30 sec.

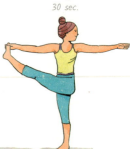

4. Revolved Chair Pose
30 sec.

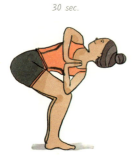

5. High Lunge w/ Arms Extended
30 sec.

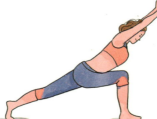

6. Easy Revolved Side Angle Pose
30 sec.

7. Revolved Side Angle Pose
30 sec.

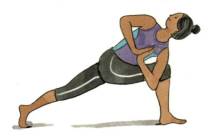

8. Downward Dog Vinyasa Flow
30 sec.

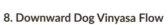
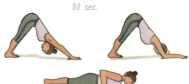
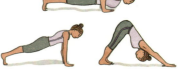

9. Four-Limbed Staff to Plank Push-Up
30-60 sec.

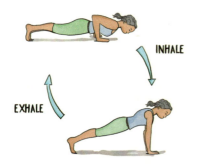

10. Child's Pose
30-60 sec.

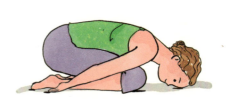

Segment 3: Cool Down

DATE

1. Thread the Needle Pose

30 sec. per side

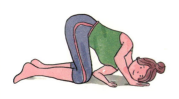

2. Striking Cobra Pose

60 sec.

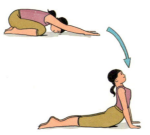

3. Easy Half Bow Pose

30 sec. per side

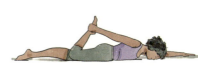

4. Half Wind Release Pose

30 sec. per side

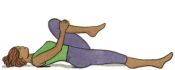

5. Happy Baby Pose

30-60 sec.

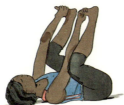

6. Supine Abdominal Twist

30 sec. per side

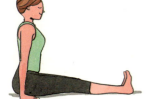

7. Staff Pose

30 sec.

8. Bharadvaja's Twist Pose

30 sec. per side

9. Easy Boat Pose

30-60 sec.

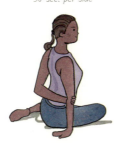
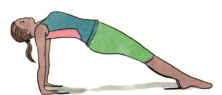

10. Upward Plank Pose
30-60 sec.

11. Corpse Pose
5 mins.

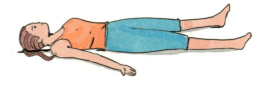

Food for Thought

Koshas: Manomaya.

The third layer of the Koshas is Manomaya Kosha, which translates to the 'mental sheath.'

It corresponds to the fire element, and it governs our thoughts, emotions, judgments, and concentration.

All of your perceptions, mental images, and inner voices come from this Kosha, as well as your opinions and core beliefs that have been shaped by your experiences.

Most of our internal beliefs and perceptions are instilled in us by the social culture we're surrounded by, so truly exploring and experimenting with those beliefs to see if they align with who we are (or want to be) can be priceless!

The best way to bring balance to this Kosha is through mindfully practicing our asanas and pranayama and making a conscious effort to positively reframe the way you think and speak about yourself and the world around you.

You can also build up this Kosha through positive affirmations and meditation!

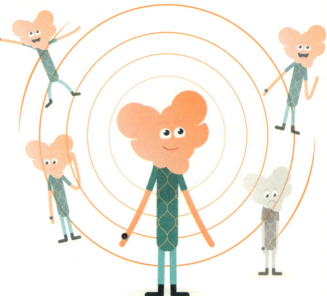

"Yoga does not remove us from the reality or responsibilities of everyday life but rather places our feet firmly and resolutely in the practical ground of experience. We don't transcend our lives; we return to the life we left behind in the hopes of something better." - Donna Farhi

Segment 1: Warm-Up

Full Session Exercise Guide:
habitnest.com/pages/yoga-day-37

1. Seated Neck Rolls
30 sec. each direction

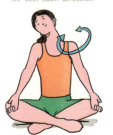

2. Seated Torso Circles
30 sec. each direction

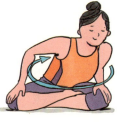

3. Cosmic Egg Pose
60 sec.

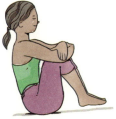

4. Seated Cat-Cow Pose
30-60 sec., alternating

5. Mountain Pose Arm Warm-Up
60 sec.

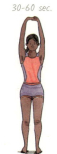

6. Palm Tree Pose
30-60 sec.

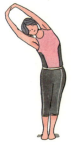

7. Palm Tree Pose w/ Side Bend
30 sec. per side

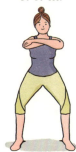

8. Standing Bound Rising Locust Pose
30-60 sec.

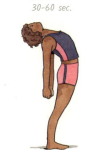

9. Standing Pelvic Circles
30 sec. each direction

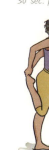

10. Standing Quad Stretch
30 sec. per side

11. Squat w/ Arms Crossed
30-60 sec.

12. Side Lunge Pose
30 sec. per side

13. Chair Pose
30 sec.

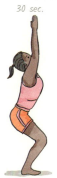

14. Half Forward Fold Pose
30-60 sec.

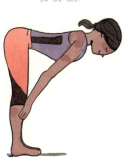

Segment 2: Peak Flow

> Repeat poses 1-12, switching to the opposite side as necessary for asymmetrical poses.

1. Five-Pointed Star Pose
30 sec.

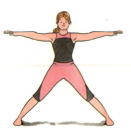

2. Triangle Pose
30 sec.

3. Revolved Triangle Pose
30 sec.

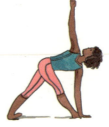

4. Extended Side Angle Pose
30 sec.

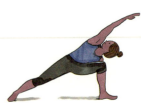

5. Easy Revolved Side Angle Pose
30 sec.

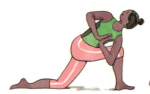

6. Intense Leg Stretch Pose I
30 sec.

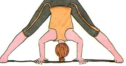

7. Intense Leg Stretch Pose II
30 sec.

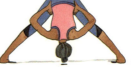

8. Intense Leg Stretch Pose III
30 sec.

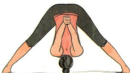

9. Intense Leg Stretch Pose IV
30 sec.

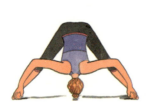

10. Warrior I Pose
30 sec.

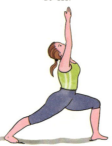

11. Warrior II Pose
30 sec.

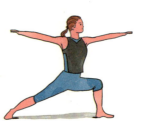

12. Goddess Pose
30-45 sec.

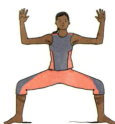

13. Wide-Legged Vinyasa Flow
30-60 sec.

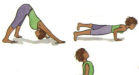

14. Frog Pose
30 sec.

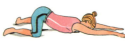

15. Locust Pose
30-60 sec.

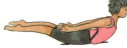

16. Crocodile Pose
30 sec.

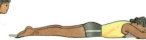

Segment 3: Cool Down

DATE

1. Locust to Wide-Legged Chariot Flow
60–90 sec.

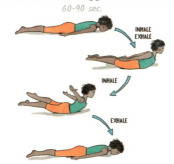

2. Crocodile Pose
30 sec.

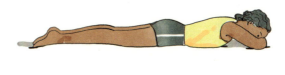

3. Downward-Facing Dog Pose
30 sec.

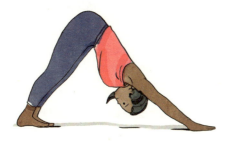

4. Sleeping Swan Pose
30 sec. per side

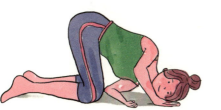

5. Thread the Needle Pose
30 sec. per side

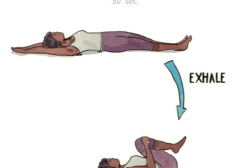

6. Reclined Leg Stretch Flow
30 sec. per side

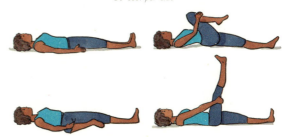

7. Full-Body Stretch to Wind Release Flow
30 sec.

8. Corpse Pose
5 mins.

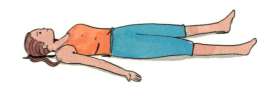

Favorite Resources

Resources: Yoga With Adriene (YT channel).

Yoga by Adriene is a great channel on YouTube for yoga practitioners at any level! Her signature phrase is to *"find what feels good,"* placing an emphasis on listening to and trusting your body.

She has uploaded tons of high-quality videos that teach core concepts of yoga, guide you through flows for all levels and body types, and meditations.

The guided flows range from under 10 minutes to an hour, providing plenty of options to fit your preferences and schedule.

Some of the flows specifically target mental health as well, which is great for aligning the energies within your subtle body (such as your Kaphas, Doshas, and Chakras) and improving your overall mental well-being.

Adriene's soothing voice and guiding cues are especially helpful for those who struggle with form and alignment without being overly distracting.

You can find Adriene's channel by heading over to YouTube and searching *"Yoga by Adriene"*!

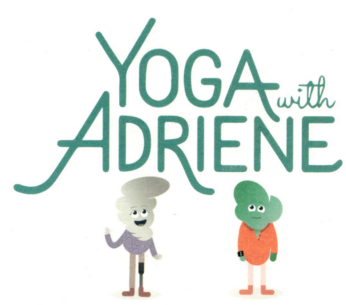

"The awesome in me bows to the awesome in you." - Adriene Mishler

Segment 1: Warm-Up

Full Session Exercise Guide:
habitnest.com/pages/yoga-day-38

1. Revolved Staff Pose Flow
30-60 sec., alternating

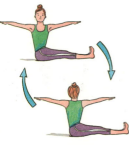

2. Seated Ankle Rotation
30 sec. each direction

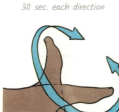

3. Seated Knee Rotation
30 sec. per side

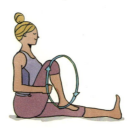

4. Seated Hip Rotation
30 sec. per side

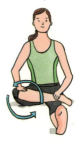

5. Shoulder Socket Rotation
30-60 sec.

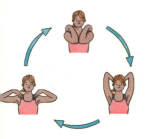

6. Neck Rolls
30 sec. each direction

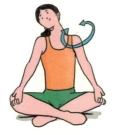

7. Easy Pose Mudra Flow
30 sec.

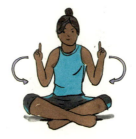

8. Wrist Rolls w/ Hands Clasped
30 sec.

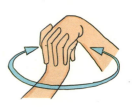

9. Easy Pose Bound Arm Rolls
30-60 sec.

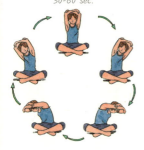

10. Easy Pose w/ Bound Hands
30-60 sec.

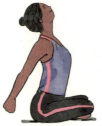

11. Easy Pose Forward Fold
30-60 sec.

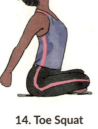

12. Cat-Cow Rib Circles
30 sec. each direction

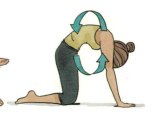

13. Table Top Pose Wrist Stretch
30-60 sec.

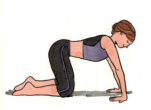

14. Toe Squat
30-60 sec.

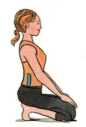

15. Thunderbolt Pose Ankle Stretch
30-60 sec.

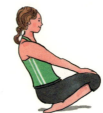

16. Spinal Rock Pose
30-60 sec.

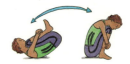

Segment 2: Peak Flow

> Repeat poses 1-8, switching to the opposite side as necessary for asymmetrical poses.

1. Wind Release to Mountain Pose Flow
30-60 sec.

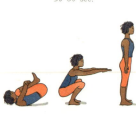

2. Mountain Pose Tiptoes Flow
30 sec.

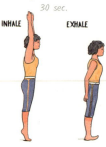

3. Chair Pose
30 sec.

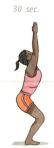

4. Standing Roll-Up Flow
60 sec.

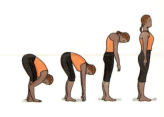

5. Chair to Revolved Chair Pose Flow
30 sec.

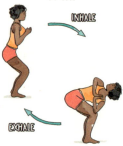

6. Warrior I w/ Cactus Arms Flow
30 sec.

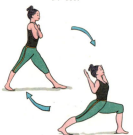

7. Reverse Warrior Pose
30 sec.

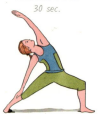

8. Triangle Pose
30 sec.

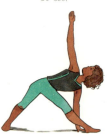

9. Warrior II to Five Pointed Star Flow
60-90 sec.

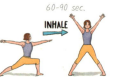
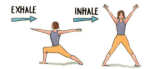

10. Intense Leg Stretch Pose
60 sec.

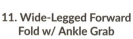

11. Wide-Legged Forward Fold w/ Ankle Grab
30 sec. per side

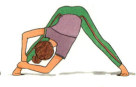

12. Mountain Pose Namaste
30 sec.

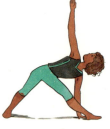

13. Extended Mountain Pose w/ Hands Interlocked
30 sec.

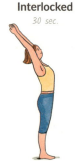

14. Upward Salute to Forward Fold Flow
60 sec.

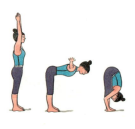

15. Plank to Downward Dog Pose Flow
60 sec.

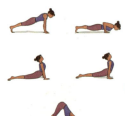

16. Thunderbolt to Child's Pose Flow
60-90 sec.

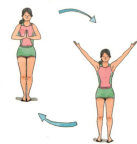

Segment 3: Cool Down

DATE

1. Camel Pose w/ Hands to Floor
30 sec.

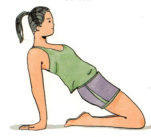

2. Puppy Dog Pose
30-60 sec.

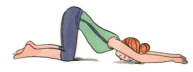

3. Reclined Hero Pose
60 sec.

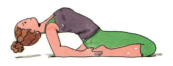

4. Child's Pose
30-60 sec.

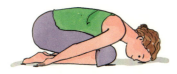

5. Table Top Pose
30-60 sec.

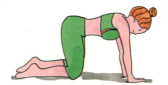

6. Crocodile Pose
30 sec.

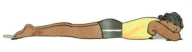

7. Sphinx Pose
60 sec.

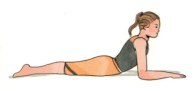

8. Reclining Bound Angle Pose
60 sec.

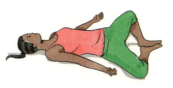

9. Happy Baby Pose
30-60 sec.

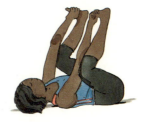

10. Half Wind Release Pose
30 sec. per side

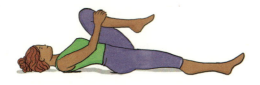

11. Corpse Pose
5 mins.

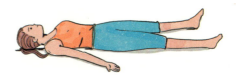

Food for Thought

Yamas: Brahmacharya (non-excess).

Though Brahmacharya is often translated as 'non-excess', 'celibacy', and 'chastity,' it doesn't refer only to your intimate energy.

Brahmacharya includes abstaining from external desires and temptations, which only offer temporary, fleeting satisfaction.

It's about using our energy in a way that leads us to a connection with our inner divinity and helps us find peace within ourselves.

The best way to evaluate and implement Brahmacharya is to ask yourself where you're directing your energy, and whether that direction is harmful or helpful to your practice.

Are you doing what you can to be the best version of yourself? Are you using your energy in a positive, impactful way, or are you wasting your energy on external temptations that provide immediate, but ultimately transient, rewards?

Take a moment to consider where you're directing your energy and how you can adjust your energy direction and behavior in a more positive direction!

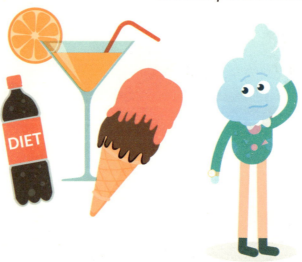

"For many years I mistook discipline as ambition. Now I believe it to be more about consistency. Do get on the mat. Practice and life are not that different." - Judith Hanson Lasater

Segment 1: Warm-Up

Full Session Exercise Guide:
habitnest.com/pages/yoga-day-39

1. Wrist Flexion/ Extension
30 sec.

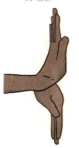

2. Wrist Rotations
30 sec.

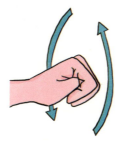

3. Neck Twists
30 sec., alternating sides

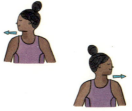

4. Standing Ankle Rotation
30 sec. per side

5. Standing Knee Rotation
30 sec. per side

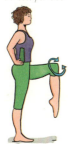

6. Leg Kicks Flow
30 sec. per side

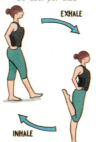

7. Side Lunge Pose w/ Arms Raised
30 sec. per side

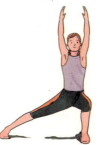

8. Standing Pelvic Circles
30 sec. each direction

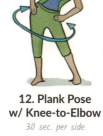

9. Intense Side Stretch
30 sec. per side

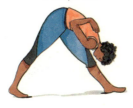

10. Standing Backbend Pose
60 sec.

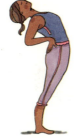

11. Standing Forward Fold Pose
30 sec.

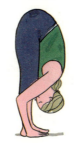

12. Plank Pose w/ Knee-to-Elbow
30 sec. per side

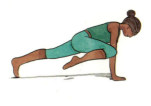

13. Forearm Plank Flow
60 sec.

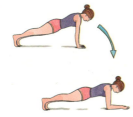

14. Forearm Plank Hip Twists
60 sec., alternating sides

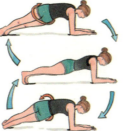

15. Sphinx Pose
60 sec.

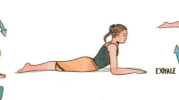

16. Sphinx Pose Cat-Cow Flow
60 sec.

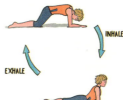

Segment 2: Peak Flow

> Repeat poses 1-7 & 9-12, switching to the opposite side as necessary for asymmetrical poses.

1. Downward-Facing Dog Pose
30 sec.

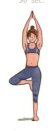

2. Downward Dog Plank Flow
30 sec.

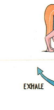

3. Forward Fold Flow
30 sec.

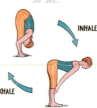

4. Volcano Pose
30 sec.

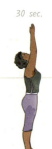

5. Tree Pose
30 sec.

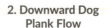

6. Dancer Pose
30 sec.

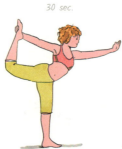

7. Warrior I Pose
30 sec.

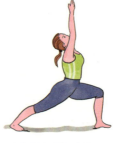

8. Downward Dog to Mountain Pose Flow
30-45 sec.

9. Downward-Facing Dog Pose
30 sec.

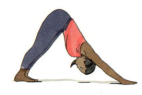

10. Plank Pose
30 sec.

11. Side Plank Pose
30 sec.

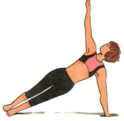

12. Wild Thing Pose
30 sec.

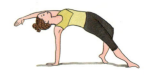

13. Wide Child's Pose
30 sec.

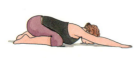

14. Eight-Limbed Striking Cobra Flow
30 sec.

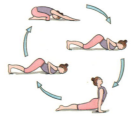

15. Puppy Dog Pose
30-60 sec.

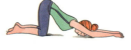

16. Child's Pose
30-60 sec.

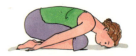

Segment 3: Cool Down

DATE

1. Bound Angle Pose
60 sec.

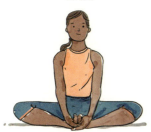

2. Seated Star Pose
60 sec.

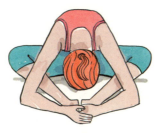

3. Half Lord of the Fishes Pose
30 sec. per side

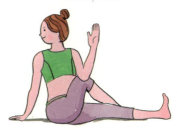

4. Sitting Swan Pose
30 sec. per side

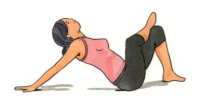

5. Happy Baby Pose
30-60 sec.

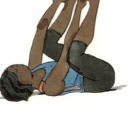

6. Supine Spinal Twist II Pose
30 sec. per side

7. Half Plow Pose
30-60 sec.

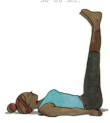

8. Fish Pose
60 sec.

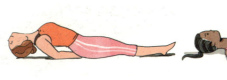

9. Reclining Bound Angle
30-60 sec.

10. Full-Body Stretch Pose
30 sec.

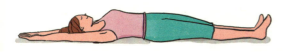

11. Corpse Pose
5 mins.

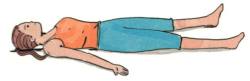

Food for Thought

Niyamas: Svadhyaya (self-study).

Svādhyāya is all about studying yourself, as well as the study of ancient yogic scriptures, such as the Bhagavad Gita, the Vedas, or Patañjali's Sutras. It's about staying curious, being receptive to new teachings, and craving to know more!

If you choose not to study the ancient texts themselves, reading up about the various topics within yoga is a sufficient alternative.

Regardless of how much you read and learn, it's all pointless until you take the time to reflect on it and figure out how that information applies to your practice.

In the process, you learn who you are, who you're not, and who you want to be. The more we understand who we are on the mat, the better we understand who we are off the mat.

You can cultivate this self-awareness throughout the day as well. Observe your actions, and ask yourself why you're doing what you're doing. Learn about your driving motivations, your sore spots, and everything that makes you tick.

Get to know and understand yourself on a whole new level, and use that to carve out a successful yoga practice!

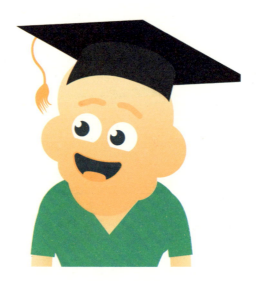

"Yoga is the journey of the self, through the self, to the Self" – The Bhagavad Gita

Segment 1: Warm-Up

Full Session Exercise Guide:
habitnest.com/pages/yoga-day-40

1. Thunderbolt Pose
30-60 sec.

2. Revolved Thunderbolt Pose
30 sec. per side

3. Kneeling Side Bends
30 sec. per side

4. Cat-Cow Pose
30-60 sec., alternating

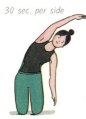
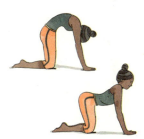

5. Child's Pose Sphinx Flow
30-60 sec.

6. Wide Child's Pose
30-60 sec.

7. Wide-Legged Vinyasa Flow
30-60 sec.

8. Downward Dog to Mountain Pose Flow
30 sec.

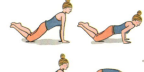
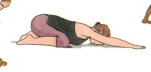

9. Mountain Pose Tiptoes Flow
30 sec.

10. Standing Arm Circles
30 sec. each direction

11. Easy Joint Warm-Up Flow
1-2 mins.

12. Mountain Pose Forward Fold Arm Swings
30 sec.

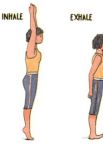
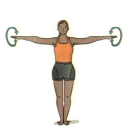
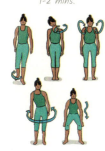
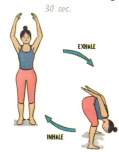

13. Standing Wind Release Pose
30 sec. per side

14. Standing Quad Stretch
30 sec. per side

15. Mountain Pose Namaste
30 sec.

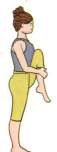
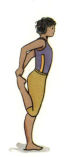
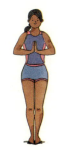

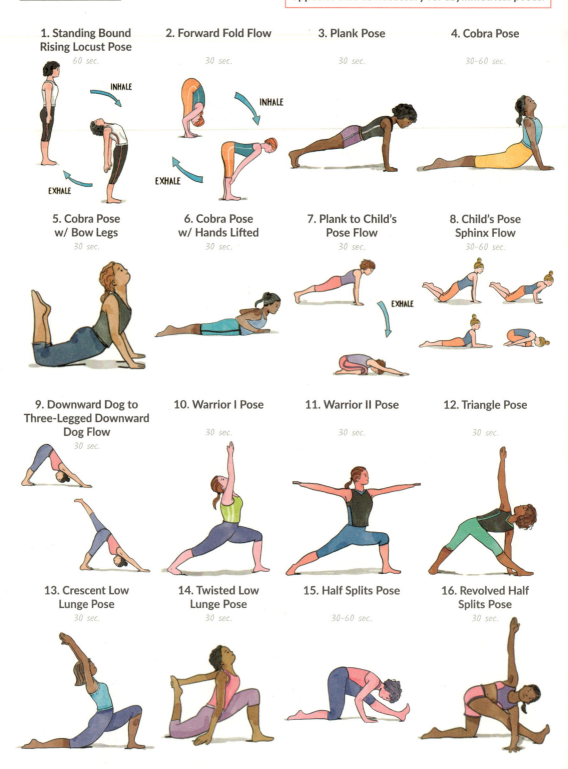

Segment 3: Cool Down

DATE

1. Downward-Facing Dog Pose
30 sec.

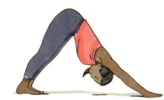

2. Pigeon Pose
30 sec. per side

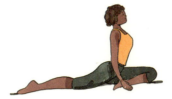

3. Sleeping Swan Pose
30-60 sec. per side

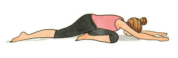

4. Revolved Pigeon Pose
30 sec. per side

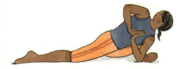

5. Head-to-Knee Pose
30 sec. per side

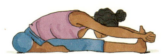

6. Revolved Head-to-Knee Pose
30 sec. per side

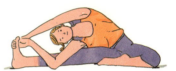

7. Bridge Pose
30-60 sec.

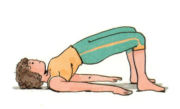

8. One-Legged Bridge Pose
30 sec. per side

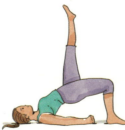

9. Happy Baby Pose
30-60 sec.

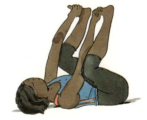

10. Supine Spinal Twist II Pose
30 sec. per side

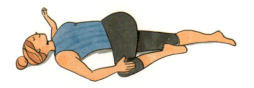

11. Corpse Pose
5 mins.

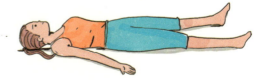

Pro-Tip

Asanas: Yin yoga tips for restorative/healing benefits.

Yin yoga (not to be confused with Restorative yoga) involves staying in postures for prolonged periods of time.

Holding the poses eventually creates some uncomfortable sensations, emotions, or thoughts that have been tucked away and stored in your muscles.

The stillness of the body helps to promote the stillness of the mind, helping you to build up stronger mental stability and resilience. Eventually, the tension in the muscles finally releases, allowing the discomfort and emotions to dissipate.

Try holding some of the postures longer during your next session.

Pay close attention to the sensations and emotions. Stay strong and push your way through that initial discomfort. Don't let your mind get caught up in the details of how the stress or tension got there, just stay focused on the pose, your breathing, and the sensations that arise.

If you move into a pose or stretch that's actually painful, don't stay in it! Release from the pose slowly and move on to a different pose.

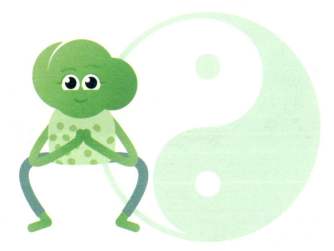

"Yoga is the ultimate practice. It simultaneously stimulates our inner light and quiets our overactive minds. It is both energy and rest. Yin and Yang. We feel the burn and find our bliss." - Elise Joan

Segment 1: Warm-Up

Full Session Exercise Guide:
habitnest.com/pages/yoga-day-41

1. Reclining Bound Angle Pose
60 sec.

2. Revolved Abdomen Twist Pose
30 sec. per side

3. Forward-to-Backward Neck Stretch
30 sec., alternating

4. Side-to-Side Neck Stretches
30 sec. per side

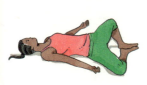 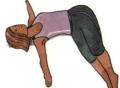

5. Alternating Shoulder Shrugs
30 sec.

6. Seated Torso Circles
30 sec. each direction

7. Seated Forward Fold Prep
60 sec.

8. Seated Straddle Prep
30-60 sec.

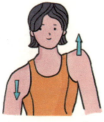 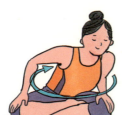 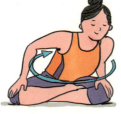 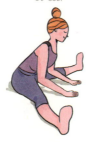 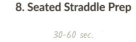

9. Sage Marichi Pose C
30 sec. per side

10. Seated Forward Fold Pose
60 sec.

11. Upward Facing Seated Straddle w/ Toe Grab
30-60 sec.

12. Cat-Cow Pose
30-60 sec., alternating

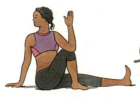 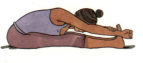 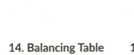 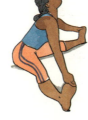 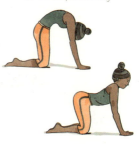

13. Table Top Side-to-Side Flow
30-60 sec.

14. Balancing Table Top Knee-to-Nose Flow
30 sec. per side

15. Unilateral Balancing Table Top Pose
30 sec. per side

16. Wide Child's Pose
30-60 sec.

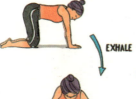 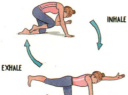 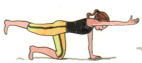 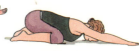

Segment 2: Peak Flow

> Repeat poses 1-8, switching to the opposite side as necessary for asymmetrical poses.

1. Standing Wind Release Pose
30 sec.

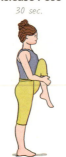

2. Tree Pose
30 sec.

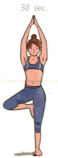

3. Revolved Hand-to-Big-Toe Pose
30 sec.

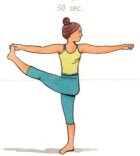

4. Revolved Chair Pose
30 sec.

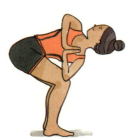

5. High Lunge w/ Arms Extended
30 sec.

6. Easy Revolved Side Angle Pose
30 sec.

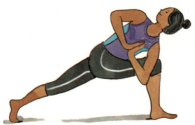

7. Revolved Side Angle Pose
30 sec.

8. Downward Dog Vinyasa Flow
30-60 sec.

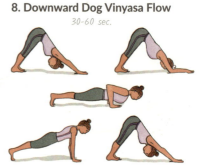

9. Four-Limbed Staff to Plank Push-Up
30-60 sec.

10. Child's Pose
30-60 sec.

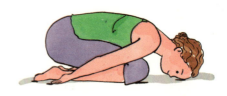

Segment 3: Cool Down

DATE

1. Bound Angle Pose
60 sec.

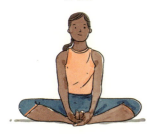

2. Seated Star Pose
60 sec.

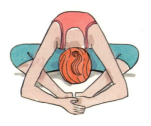

3. Half Lord of the Fishes Pose
30 sec. per side

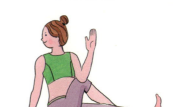

4. Sitting Swan Pose
30 sec. per side

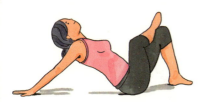

5. Happy Baby Pose
30-60 sec.

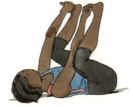

6. Supine Spinal Twist II Pose
30 sec. per side

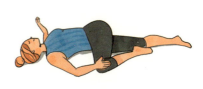

7. Half Plow Pose
30-60 sec.

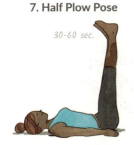

8. Fish Pose
60 sec.

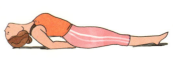

9. Reclining Bound Angle Pose
30-60 sec.

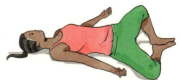

10. Full-Body Stretch Pose
30-60 sec.

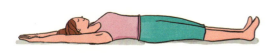

11. Corpse Pose
5 mins.

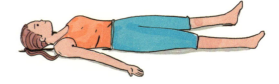

Actionable Challenge

Pranayama: Bumble Bee Breath.

Bumble Bee Breath, or Bhramari Pranayama, is an easy, effective breathing technique to help you reduce distractions and direct your concentration.

Bumble Bee Breath is great for clearing up respiratory congestion and getting your blood circulating, and it's even a fun and easy method to do with kids! It also helps reduce stress and regulate your nervous system.

This super simple breathing exercise can be performed anywhere, so give it a shot sometime today when you need to restore your focus or eliminate distractions!

All you have to do for this breathing practice is to keep your mouth closed, take a deep inhale, then hum as you exhale, creating one continuous humming tone the entire time. The humming should resemble the sound of a buzzing bumblebee.

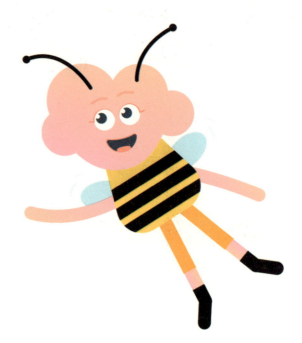

Actionable Challenge Completed: ☐

"At this moment, you are seamlessly flowing with the cosmos. There is no difference between your breathing and the breathing of the rainforest, between your bloodstream and the world's rivers, between your bones and the chalk cliffs of Dover."- Deepak Chopra

Segment 1: Warm-Up

Full Session Exercise Guide:
habitnest.com/pages/yoga-day-42

1. Three-Part Breath
2 mins.

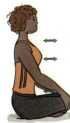

2. Seated Neck Rolls
30 sec. each direction

3. Wrist Rolls w/ Hands Clasped
30 sec.

4. Seated Torso Circles
30 sec. each direction

5. Seated Butterfly Pose Wings
60 sec.

6. Fish Pose w/ Butterfly Legs
60 sec.

7. Bound Angle Upward Plank Pose Flow
30-60 sec.

8. Seated Star Pose
60 sec.

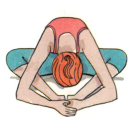

9. Thread the Needle Pose Flow
30 sec. per side

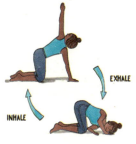

10. Table Top Pose w/ Knee Lift
30 sec.

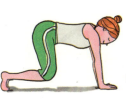

11. Table Top Pose Lifted Knee Cat-Cow Flow
30 sec.

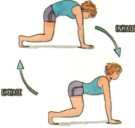

12. Downward-Facing Dog Pose
30-60 sec.

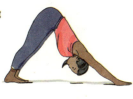

13. Dangling Pose
60 sec.

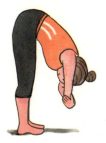

14. Standing Roll-Up Flow
30 sec.

15. Sun Salutation Variation A
~1-2 mins.

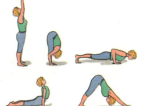

16. Sun Salutation Variation B
~1-2 mins.

Segment 2: Peak Flow

> Repeat poses 1-8, switching to the opposite side as necessary for asymmetrical poses.

1. Mountain Pose
30 sec.

2. One-Legged Mountain Pose w/ Side Bend
30 sec.

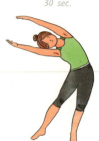

3. Chair Pose
30 sec.

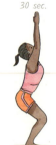

4. Revolved Chair Pose
30 sec.

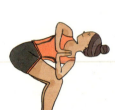

5. Vinyasa I
30 sec.

6. Reverse Warrior Pose
30 sec.

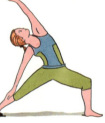

7. Twisted Reverse Warrior Pose
30 sec.

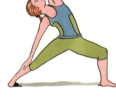

8. Extended Side Angle Pose
30 sec.

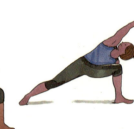

9. Standing Forward Fold Pose
30-60 sec.

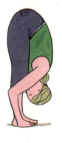

10. Crow Pose w/ Toe Taps
30 sec. per side

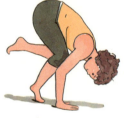

11. Plank Pose
30 sec.

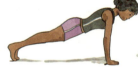

12. Child's Pose
30-60 sec.

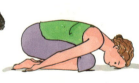

13. Rabbit Pose
30-60 sec.

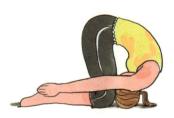

14. Toe Squat Pose w/ Cat-Cow Flow
30-60 sec.

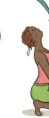

INHALE

EXHALE

15. Thunderbolt Pose Heart Opener
60 sec.

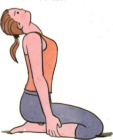

Segment 3: Cool Down

DATE

1. Child's Pose

30-60 sec.

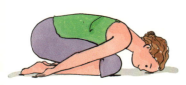

2. Half Lord of the Fishes Pose

30 sec. per side

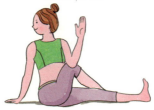

3. Staff Pose w/ Feet Movements

30 sec.

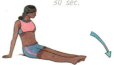
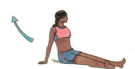
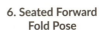

4. Staff Pose w/ Hands Back

30 sec.

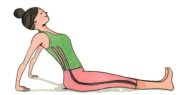

5. Upward Plank Pose

30-60 sec.

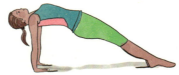

6. Seated Forward Fold Pose

60 sec.

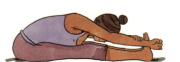

7. Wind Release Pose

60 sec.

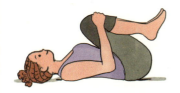

8. Bridge Pose

30-60 sec.

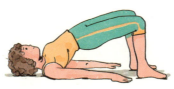

9. Supine Spinal Twist II Pose

30 sec. per side

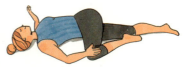

10. Happy Baby Pose

30-60 sec.

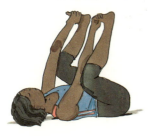

11. Reclining Bound Angle Pose w/ Elbow Grab

30-60 sec.

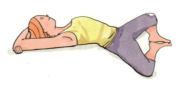

12. Corpse Pose

5 mins.

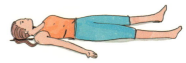

Food for Thought

Pratyahara: pushing through times you "don't feel like it."

Everyone encounters 'off days' - days when they lack motivation, don't feel up to the task, or are simply too busy. This is completely normal and expected. The likelihood that you'll practice yoga every single day for the rest of your life is pretty low, so don't sweat it if you fall off track.

The important thing is that you pick it back up the next day. Don't let a one-day break turn into a week, a month, or a year of skipping your routine.

Once you fall off track, it's easy for your mind to form the counterproductive belief that it's okay to miss your flow again, or make unconscious decisions to justify missing it.

Instead of beating yourself up on these days, cherish them and push through them to stay consistent! Vow to return to your habit the next day, and hold yourself accountable for sticking to it and doing what you say you'll do.

You've made it this far already, and your practice has come so far since Day 1.

Celebrate your progress - you're an absolute warrior for working so hard at this! Keep on keeping on, and pay no mind to those 'off' days. Allow them to pass, then move on from them.

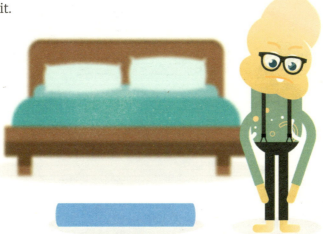

"If you fall over, you fall over. If you have to stop, you stop. But you start again. Just like life itself, you start again." - Gurmukh Kaur Khalsa

Segment 1: Warm-Up

Full Session Exercise Guide:
habitnest.com/pages/yoga-day-43

1. Alternate Nostril Breathing
2 mins.

2. Easy Pose Warm-Up
1-2 mins.

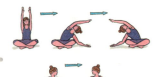

3. Seated Neck Rolls
30 sec. each direction

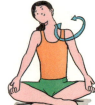

4. Neck Twists
30 sec. each direction

5. Side-to-Side Neck Stretch
30 sec. each side

6. Forward-to-Backward Neck Stretch
30 sec. each direction

7. Cat-Cow Pose w/ Lateral Leg Extension
30 sec. per side

8. Tiger Pose Crunches
30 sec. per side

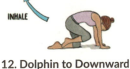

9. Table Top Pose Wrist Stretch
30 sec.

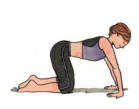

10. Child's Pose Cat-Cow Flow
60 sec.

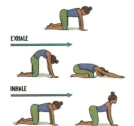

11. Thread the Needle Pose Flow
30 sec. per side

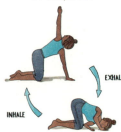

12. Dolphin to Downward Dog Push-Ups
30-60 sec.

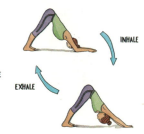

13. Half Headstand Pose
30-60 sec.

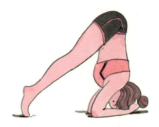

14. Tripod Pose Prep
30 sec. per side

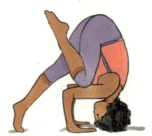

15. Crocodile Pose on Elbows
30 sec.

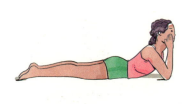

Segment 2: Peak Flow

> Repeat poses 1-8, switching to the opposite side as necessary for asymmetrical poses.

1. Mountain Pose
30 sec.

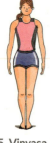

2. One-Legged Mountain Pose w/ Side Bend
30-60 sec.

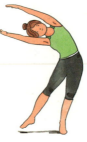

3. Chair Pose
30 sec.

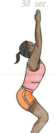

4. Revolved Chair Pose
30 sec.

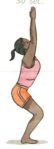

5. Vinyasa I
30 sec.

6. Reverse Warrior Pose
30 sec.

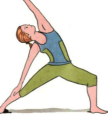

7. Twisted Reverse Warrior Pose
30 sec.

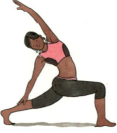

8. Extended Side Angle Pose
30 sec.

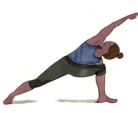

9. Standing Forward Fold Pose
30-60 sec.

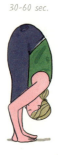

10. Crow Pose w/ Toe Taps
30 sec. per side

11. Plank Pose
30 sec.

12. Child's Pose
30-60 sec.

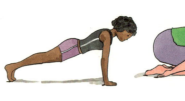

13. Rabbit Pose
30-60 sec.

14. Toe Squat Pose w/ Cat-Cow Flow
30-60 sec.

15. Thunderbolt Pose Heart Opener
60 sec.

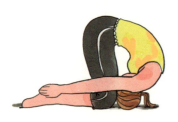

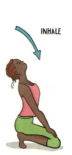

INHALE

EXHALE

Segment 3: Cool Down

DATE

1. Reclining Bound Angle Pose
60 sec.

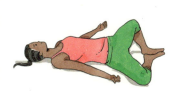

2. Supine Butterfly Wings Flow
30-60 sec.

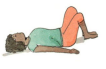
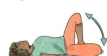

3. Banana Pose w/ Ankles Crossed
30 sec. per side

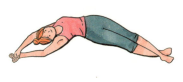

4. Wind Release Pose
60 sec.

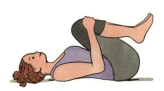

5. Supine Spinal Twist II Pose
30 sec. per side

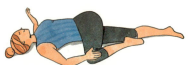

6. Happy Baby Pose
30-60 sec.

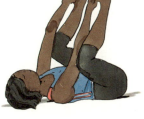

7. Reclined Cow Face Pose
30 sec., then reverse legs & repeat

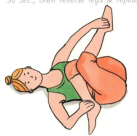

8. Cat Pulling Tail Pose
30 sec. per side

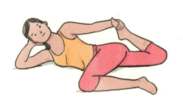

9. Supine Spinal Twist Shoulder Stretch Flow
30 sec. per side

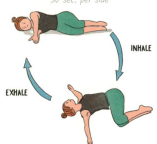

10. Crocodile Pose
30 sec.

11. Easy Half Bow Pose
30 sec. per side

12. Corpse Pose
5 mins.

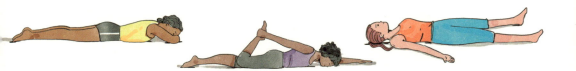

Pro-Tip

Dharana: don't compare yourself or your progress to others.

Growing and building a personal yoga practice is no easy feat. It involves a lot of dedication, openness, persistence, resilience, and progress that will never match someone else's life journey or yoga practice.

Your practice is unique to you, just as anyone else's practice is unique. Refrain from comparing your progress to anyone else's.

Your journey will never exactly match someone else's. Your body, your movements, and your flow will all be different from everyone else's.

Be mindful of your thoughts during today's practice, and if you catch yourself making comparisons, stop and remind yourself that you are exactly where you should be in your journey right now.

This isn't a competition, and comparison is the enemy of peace, contentment, and true self-acceptance.

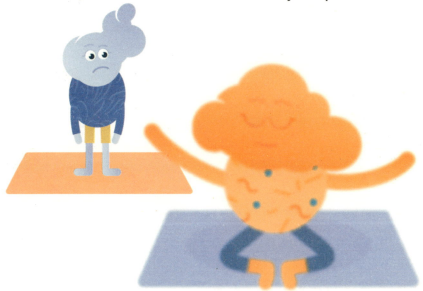

"A flower does not think of competing with the flower next to it. It just blooms."
- Zen Shin

Segment 1: Warm-Up

Full Session Exercise Guide:
habitnest.com/pages/yoga-day-44

1. Bound Angle Pose

60 sec.

2. Cradle Pose

30 sec. per side

3. Head-to-Knee Pose

30 sec. per side

4. Revolved Head-to-Knee Pose

30 sec. per side

5. Crocodile Pose

30 sec.

6. Locust Pose

30-60 sec.

7. Dolphin Pose

60 sec.

8. Three-Legged Downward-Facing Dog Pose

30 sec. per side

9. Lizard Pose

30-60 sec. per side

10. Triangle Pose w/ Bent Knee

30 sec. per side

11. Standing Forward Fold Pose

30 sec.

12. Dangling Pose

30 sec.

13. Chair Pose

30 sec.

14. Standing Backbend Pose

30-60 sec.

Segment 2: Peak Flow

> Repeat poses 1-4 & 5-8, switching to the opposite side as necessary for asymmetrical poses.

1. Tree Pose
30-60 sec.

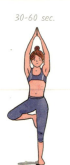

2. Tree Pose w/ Side Bends
30 sec.

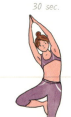

3. Chair Pose
30 sec.

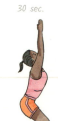

4. Revolved Chair Pose
30 sec.

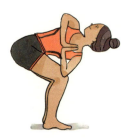

5. Downward Dog to Upward Dog Pose Flow
30 sec.

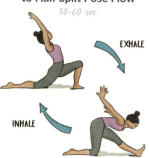

6. Three-Legged Downward-Facing Dog Pose
30 sec.

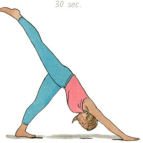

7. Bound Warrior to Humble Warrior Pose Flow
30-60 sec.

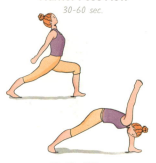

8. Crescent Low Lunge to Half Split Pose Flow
30-60 sec.

EXHALE

INHALE

9. Crow Pose w/ Toe Taps
30-60 sec. per side

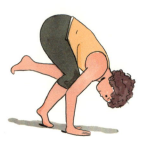

10. Staff Pose
30 sec.

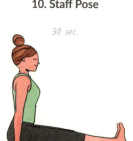

11. Seated Forward Fold Pose
60 sec.

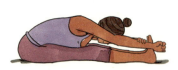

12. Wind Release Pose
60 sec.

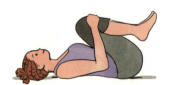

Segment 3: Cool Down

DATE

1. Reclining Bound Angle Pose
60 sec.

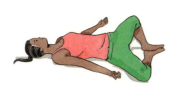

2. Supine Butterfly Wings Flow
30-60 sec.

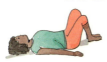
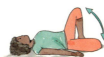

3. Banana Pose w/ Ankles Crossed
30 sec. per side

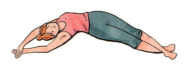

4. Wind Release Pose
60 sec.

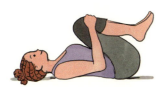

5. Supine Spinal Twist II Pose
30 sec. per side

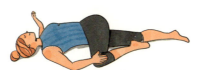

6. Happy Baby Pose
30-60 sec.

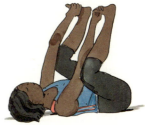

7. Reclined Cow Face Pose
30 sec., then reverse legs & repeat

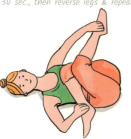

8. Cat Pulling Tail Pose
30 sec. per side

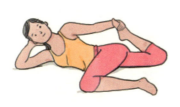

9. Supine Spinal Twist Shoulder Stretch Flow
30 sec. per side

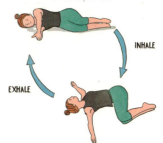
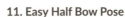

10. Crocodile Pose
30 sec.

11. Easy Half Bow Pose
30 sec. per side

12. Corpse Pose
5 mins.

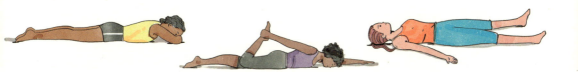

Food for Thought

Dhyana: *The Art of Stillness* **by Pico Iyer.**

This world can be incredibly demanding and taxing to our minds. In this mesmerizing TED Talk, Pico Iyer discusses the value that can be gained from setting aside time to meditate and completely still your mind.

Iyer also provides helpful strategies that anyone can implement to help us deepen our meditation and shut out the overwhelming, stressful, and distracting thoughts that try to disrupt our peace.

The talk itself creates a meditative state that brings awareness to our thoughts and concentration.

You can check out Pico's TED Talk by searching 'The Art of Stillness' on Google, YouTube, or the TED website!

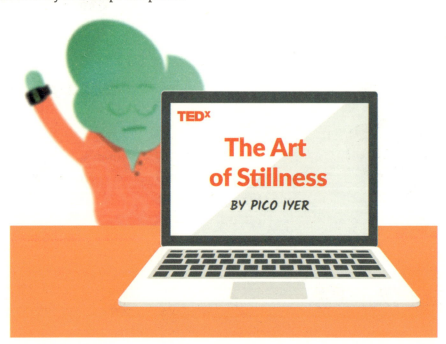

"Yoga is a way of moving into stillness in order to experience the truth of who you are." - Erich Schiffmann

Segment 1: Warm-Up

Full Session Exercise Guide:
habitnest.com/pages/yoga-day-45

1. Seated Torso Circles
30 sec. each direction

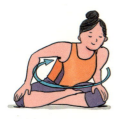

2. Shoulder Socket Rotations
30-60 sec.

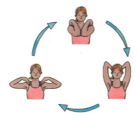

3. Revolved Easy Pose Salute Flow
60 sec., alternating sides

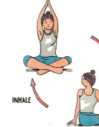

4. Easy Pose Side Bend
30 sec. per side

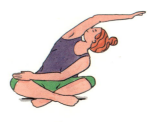

5. Seated Butterfly Pose Wings
30 sec.

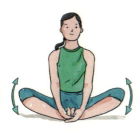

6. Bound Butterfly Wings Flow
30-60 sec.

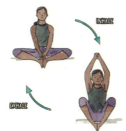

7. Fish Pose w/ Butterfly Legs
60 sec.

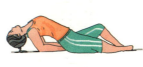

8. Seated Star Pose
60 sec.

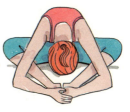

9. Table Top Pose
30 sec.

10. Table Top Pose Wrist Stretch
30 sec.

11. Cat-Cow Rib Circles
30-45 sec. each direction

12. Plank Knee-to-Nose Flow
30 sec. per side

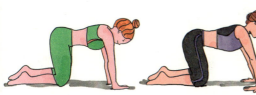
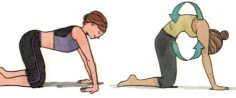
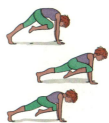

13. Reclined Single-Hip Rotations
30 sec. per side

14. Wind Release Flow
30-60 sec.

15. Half Plow to Wide-Legged Half Plow Flow
60 sec.

16. Dead Bug Core Workout I
60 sec.

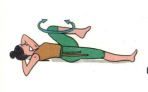
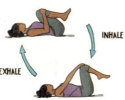
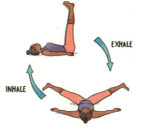
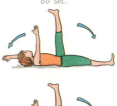
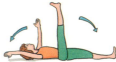

Segment 2: Peak Flow

> Repeat poses 1-4, switching to the opposite side as necessary for asymmetrical poses.

1. Plank to Downward Dog Pose Flow
30 sec.

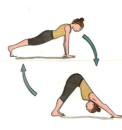

2. Three-Legged Downward Dog to Tiger Curl Flow
30 sec.

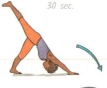

3. Lizard Pose
30-60 sec.

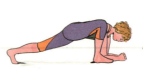

4. Pigeon Pose Forward Fold Flow
30-60 sec.

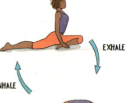

5. Plank to Downward Dog Pose Flow
30 sec.

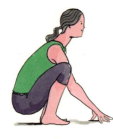

6. Standing Forward Fold Pose
30-60 sec.

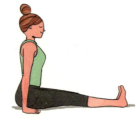

7. Extended Mountain Pose Backbend
30 sec.

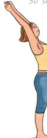

8. Mountain Pose Backbend w/ Cactus Arms
30 sec.

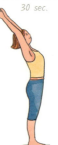

9. Garland Pose w/ Hands Forward
30 sec.

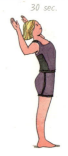

10. Staff Pose
30 sec.

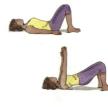

11. Bridge Pose w/ Arm Flow
30-60 sec.

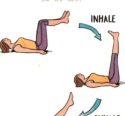

12. Half Plow Pose Flow
30-60 sec.

13. Shoulderstand Pose
30-60 sec.

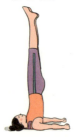

14. Wind Release Pose
60 sec.

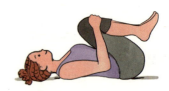

Segment 3: Cool Down

DATE

1. Fish Pose
60 sec.

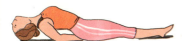

2. Full-Body Stretch Pose
60 sec.

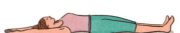

3. Half Wind Release Pose
30 sec. per side

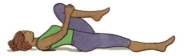

4. Wind Release Pose
60 sec.

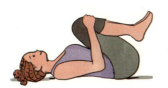

5. Scorpion Twist Pose
30 sec. per side

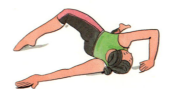

6. Supine Butterfly Pose Wings
30-60 sec.

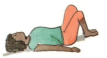
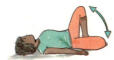

7. Supine Windshield Wipers
30 sec. per side

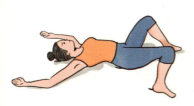

8. Reverse Pigeon Pose
30 sec. per side

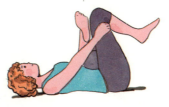

9. Reclined Half Cow Face Pose
30-60 sec. per side

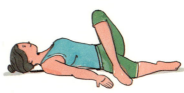

10. Reclined Cow Face Pose
30 sec., then reverse legs & repeat

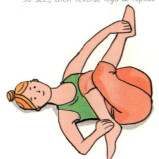

11. Corpse Pose
5 mins.

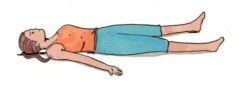

Food for Thought

Chakras: Heart Chakra (Anahata).

The Heart Chakra, located in the center of your chest, contributes to our respiration, circulation, and all of the various emotional experiences we have.

The Sanksrit word for this Chakra, Anahata, translates to 'unbroken' or 'unstuck.'

A balanced Heart Chakra can help us deepen our compassion, love, and faith in ourselves, others, or divine beings.

It can quiet the disheartening feelings of insecurity and loneliness, or it can amplify them if it's unbalanced, leading to dysfunction, distrust, and co-dependency in relationships.

This Chakra is associated with:

Color - Green

Element - Air

Sound - Yam

If your Heart Chakra is out of whack, try:

- Meditations that focus on loving-kindness
- Positive affirmations
- Practicing gratitude
- Heart-opening asanas, such as Camel Pose

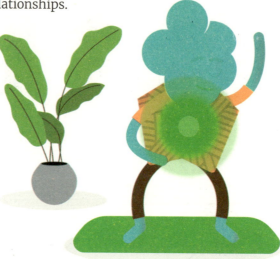

"In the chakras, it's the heart chakra, Anahata, the central chakra, three above and three below, which symbolizes happiness and love, psychic oneness, spiritual understanding." - Frederick Lenz

Segment 1: Warm-Up

Full Session Exercise Guide:
habitnest.com/pages/yoga-day-46

1. Three-Part Breath
2 mins.

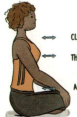

2. Seated Neck Rolls
30 sec. each direction

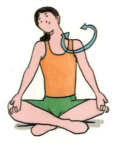

3. Wrist Rolls w/ Hands Clasped
30 sec.

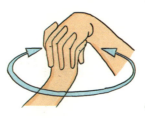

4. Seated Torso Circles
30 sec. each direction

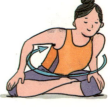

5. Seated Butterfly Pose Wings
60 sec.

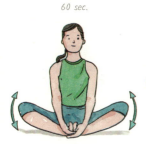

6. Fish Pose w/ Butterfly Legs
60 sec.

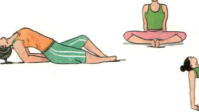

7. Bound Angle Upward Plank Pose Flow
30-60 sec.

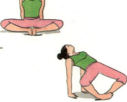

8. Seated Star Pose
60 sec.

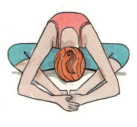

9. Thread the Needle Pose Flow
30 sec. per side

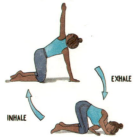

10. Table Top Pose w/ Knee Lift
30 sec.

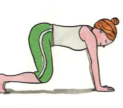

11. Table Top Pose Lifted Knee Cat-Cow Flow
30 sec.

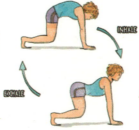

12. Downward-Facing Dog Pose
30-60 sec.

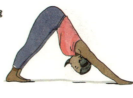

13. Dangling Pose
60 sec.

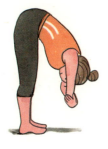

14. Standing Roll-Up Flow
30 sec.

15. Sun Salutation Variation A
1-2 mins.

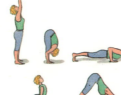

16. Sun Salutation Variation B
1-2 mins.

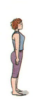

Segment 2: Peak Flow

> Repeat poses 1-12, switching to the opposite side as necessary for asymmetrical poses.

1. Five-Pointed Star Pose
30 sec.

2. Triangle Pose
30 sec.

3. Revolved Triangle Pose
30 sec.

4. Extended Side Angle Pose
30 sec.

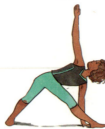

5. Easy Revolved Side Angle Pose
30 sec.

6. Intense Leg Stretch Pose I
30 sec.

7. Intense Leg Stretch Pose II
30 sec.

8. Intense Leg Stretch Pose III
30 sec.

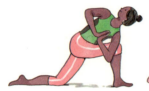 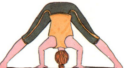 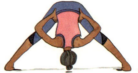 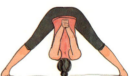

9. Intense Leg Stretch Pose IV
30 sec.

10. Warrior I Pose
30 sec.

11. Warrior II Pose
30 sec.

12. Goddess Pose
30-45 sec.

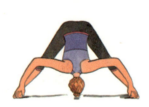 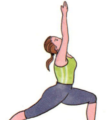 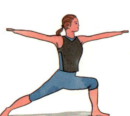

13. Wide-Legged Vinyasa Flow
30-60 sec.

14. Frog Pose
30 sec.

15. Locust Pose
30-60 sec.

16. Crocodile Pose
30 sec.

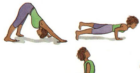 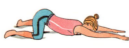 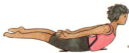 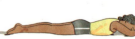

Segment 3: Cool Down

DATE

1. Bound Angle Pose
60 sec.

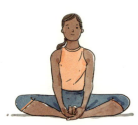

2. Seated Star Pose
60 sec.

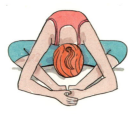

3. Fish Pose w/ Butterfly Legs
60 sec.

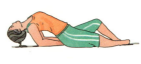

4. Staff Pose
15-30 sec.

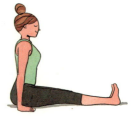

5. Half Lord of the Fishes Pose
30 sec. per side

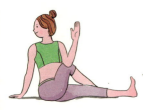

6. Seated Forward Fold Pose
60 sec.

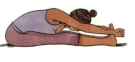

7. Upward-Facing Seated Straddle Pose
30-60 sec.

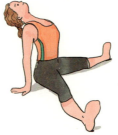

8. Revolved Head-to-Knee Pose
30 sec. per side

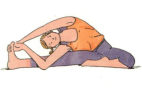

9. Bridge Pose
30-60 sec.

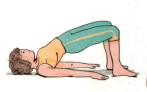

10. Staff Pose w/ Hands Back
15 sec.

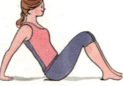

11. Reverse Table Top Pose
30 sec.

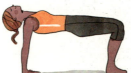

12. Reclined Hand-to-Big-Toe Pose
30 sec. per side

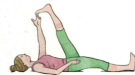

13. Reverse Pigeon Pose
30 sec. per side

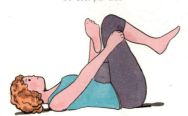

14. Corpse Pose
5 mins.

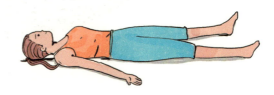

Food for Thought

Koshas: Vijnanamaya.

The fourth Kosha, Vijnanamaya, translates to our 'intellect' or 'intuitive' sheath.

This is where we store our knowledge and wisdom about ourselves and the world around us. It is our awareness of the world, our body, and how we interact.

Much like the previous Koshas, you can naturally develop your Vijnanamaya Kosha through regular asana practice, Pranayama exercises, and meditation.

Cultivate mindfulness, awareness, and even a sense of curiosity and wonder about yourself and the world around you.

These practices will carry on into your everyday life, making you more mindful and understanding of your thoughts, behaviors, and emotions. The more you understand them, the better you become at controlling them and mastering your yoga practice!

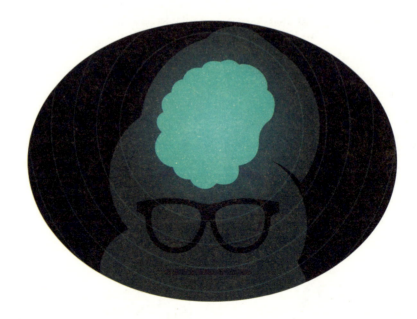

"The nature of yoga is to shine the light of awareness into the darkest corners of the body." - Jason Crandell

Segment 1: Warm-Up

Full Session Exercise Guide:
habitnest.com/pages/yoga-day-47

1. Seated Neck Rolls
30 sec. each direction

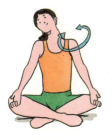

2. Easy Pose Mudra Flow
30 sec.

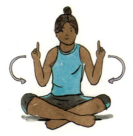

3. Seated Shoulder Rolls
30 sec. forward & backward

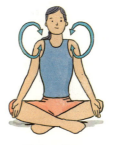

4. Cactus Arms Shoulder Movements
30-60 sec., alternating

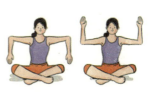

5. Deltoid Stretch
30 sec. per side

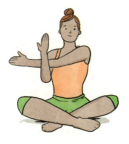

6. Side-to-Side Neck Stretch
30 sec. per side

7. Easy Pose Side Bend
30 sec. per side

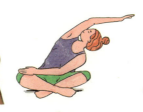

8. Revolved Easy Pose Salute Flow
30-60 sec., alternating side

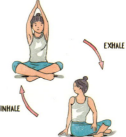

9. Seated Cat-Cow Pose
30-60 sec., alternating

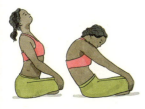

10. Staff Pose
30 sec.

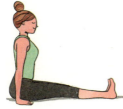

11. Seated Side Straddle Pose
30 sec. per side

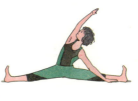

12. Upward-Facing Seated Straddle w/ Toe Grab
30-60 sec.

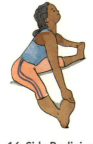

13. Seated Forward Fold Pose
60 sec.

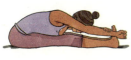

14. Supine Spinal Twist Pose
30 sec. per side

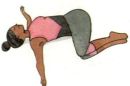

15. Side Reclining Scissors Flow
30 sec. per side

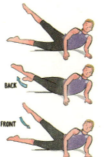

16. Side Reclining Leg Lift
30 sec. per side

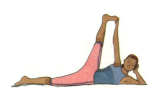

Segment 2: Peak Flow

> Repeat poses 1-8, switching to the opposite side as necessary for asymmetrical poses.

1. Downward-Facing Dog Pose
30 sec.

2. Garland Pose
30 sec.

3. Twisted Dragon Pose
30 sec.

4. Twisted Low Lunge Pose
30 sec.

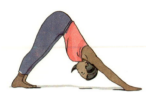
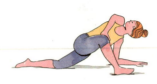
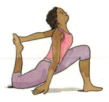

5. Warrior I Pose
30 sec.

6. Reverse Warrior Pose
30 sec.

7. Goddess Pose
30-45 sec.

8. Plank Pose
30 sec.

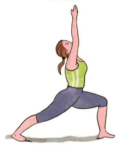
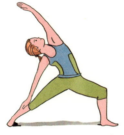
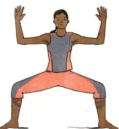
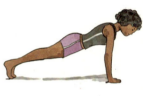

9. Full-Body Stretch Pose
30 sec.

10. Half Boat Pose
30-60 sec.

11. Constructive Rest Pose
30-60 sec.

12. Bridge Pose w/ Arm Flow
30-60 sec.

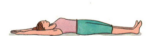
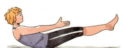
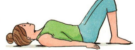

13. Supine Spinal Twist Pose
30 sec. per side

14. Reclined Hand-to-Big-Toe Pose
30 sec. per side

15. Happy Baby Pose
30-60 sec.

16. Reclining Bound Angle Pose
30-60 sec.

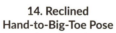

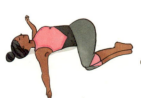
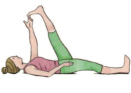
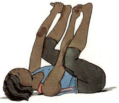
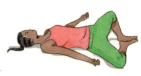

Segment 3: Cool Down

DATE

1. Seated Star Pose

60 sec.

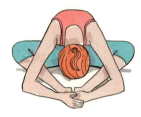

2. Head-to-Knee Pose

30 sec. per side

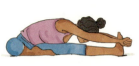

3. Boat Pose w/ Knees Bent

30 sec.

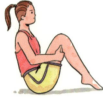

Remember not to tuck the chin too much. Keep core engaged.

4. Easy Boat Pose

30-60 sec.

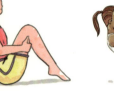

5. Staff Pose w/ Hands Back

30 sec.

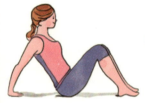

6. Reverse Table Top Pose

30 sec.

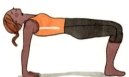

7. Caterpillar Pose

30-60 sec.

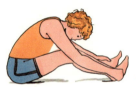

8. Supine Knee Circles

30 sec. each direction

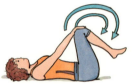

9. Half Wind Release Leg Raise Flow

30 sec. per side

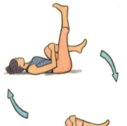
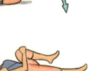

10. Supine Spinal Twist II Pose

30 sec. per side

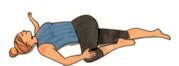

11. Supine Tree Pose

30 sec. per side

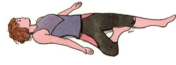

12. Full-Body Stretch w/ Gesture of the Pond

30-60 sec.

INHALE

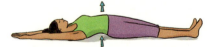

EXHALE

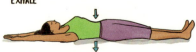

13. Corpse Pose

5 mins.

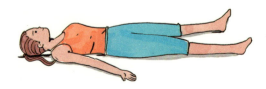

Food for Thought

Doshas: Vata.

The last of the Doshas, Vata, translates from Sanskrit to 'wind'. Appropriately, this Dosha controls your circulation, respiration, and flow of movements.

Without properly balancing Vata, you cannot create stability for the other 2 Doshas. Vata is a vital piece of the puzzle for mastering your Doshas!

An imbalance of this Dosha often leads to anxiety, poor sleep, irregular digestion, trouble keeping the mind and body still, and erratic behavior.

The Kapha and Pitta Doshas crumble without it, inevitably throwing off your entire energy balance.

Vata is best promoted through soothing routines and rituals.

Whether it's a pre-bedtime ritual, a morning routine, or just your daily yoga practice, incorporate some soothing massages, breathwork, grounding exercises, and calming music!

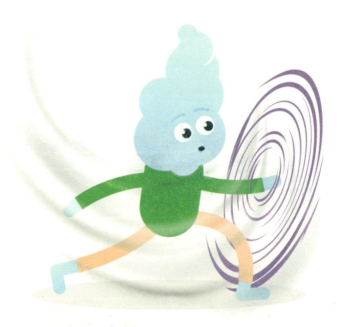

"If you seek peace, be still. If you seek wisdom, be silent. If you seek love, be yourself." - Becca Lee

Segment 1: Warm-Up

Full Session Exercise Guide:
habitnest.com/pages/yoga-day-48

1. Alternate Nostril Breathing
2 mins.

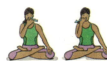

2. Easy Pose Warm-Up
1-2 mins.

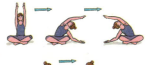

3. Seated Neck Rolls
30 sec. each direction

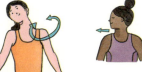

4. Neck Twists
30 sec. each direction

5. Side-to-Side Neck Stretch
30 sec. per side

6. Forward-to-Backward Neck Stretch
30 sec. each direction

7. Cat-Cow Pose w/ Lateral Leg Extension
30 sec. per side

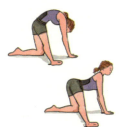

8. Tiger Pose Crunches
30 sec. per side

9. Table Top Pose Wrist Stretch
30 sec.

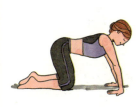

10. Child's Pose Cat-Cow Flow
60 sec.

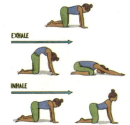

11. Thread the Needle Pose Flow
30 sec. per side

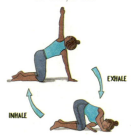

12. Dolphin to Downward Dog Push-Ups
30-60 sec.

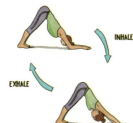

13. Half Headstand Pose
30-60 sec.

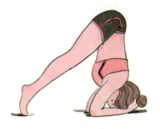

14. Tripod Pose Prep
30 sec. per side

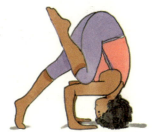

15. Crocodile Pose on Elbows
30 sec.

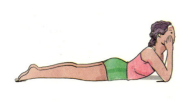

Segment 2: Peak Flow

Repeat poses 1-12, switching to the opposite side as necessary for asymmetrical poses.

1. **Downward Dog to Three-Legged Downward Dog Pose Flow** *30-60 sec.*
2. **Fallen Triangle Pose** *30 sec.*
3. **Runner's Lunge Pose** *30 sec.*
4. **Triangle Pose Side Stretch** *30 sec.*
5. **Warrior II Pose** *30 sec.*
6. **Downward Dog to Three-Legged Downward Dog Pose Flow** *30 sec.*
7. **Low Lunge Pose** *30 sec.*
8. **Low Lunge w/ Tricep Stretch** *30 sec.*
9. **High Lunge Pose** *30 sec.*
10. **Revolved High Lunge Pose** *30 sec.*
11. **Side Lunge Pose** *30 sec.*
12. **Wide-Legged Lateral Squat** *30 sec.*
13. **Plank Pose** *30 sec.*
14. **Vinyasa II** *60 sec.*
15. **Thunderbolt Pose** *30-60 sec.*

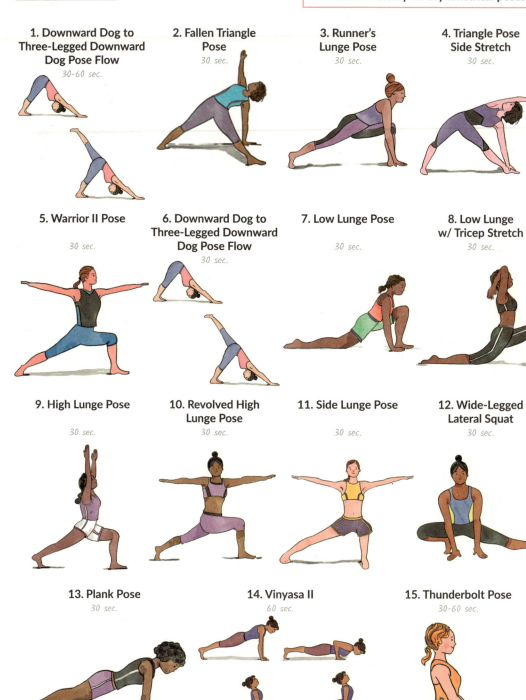

Segment 3: Cool Down

DATE

1. Camel Pose w/ Hands to Floor
30 sec.

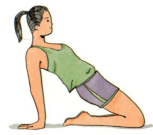

2. Puppy Dog Pose
30-60 sec.

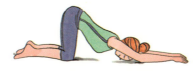

3. Reclined Hero Pose
60 sec.

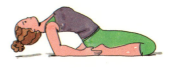

4. Child's Pose
30-60 sec.

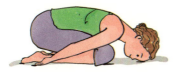

5. Table Top Pose
30-60 sec.

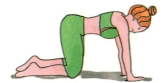

6. Crocodile Pose
30 sec.

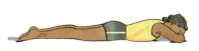

7. Sphinx Pose
60 sec.

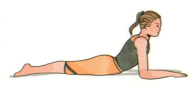

8. Reclining Bound Angle Pose
60 sec.

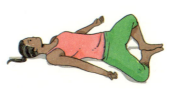

9. Happy Baby Pose
30-60 sec.

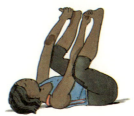

10. Half Wind Release Pose
30 sec. per side

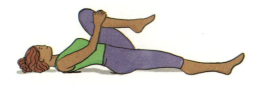

11. Corpse Pose
5 mins.

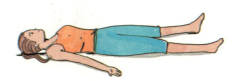

Food for Thought

Yamas: Aparigraha (non-possessiveness).

Similar to Asteya, Aparigraha is all about getting rid of your greed, jealousy, and the desire to accumulate material items.

It challenges you to sever your attachment to the material world by focusing on obtaining only the necessities of life.

Ultimately, Aparigraha is about taking only what you need, and nothing more. It can also simply mean that you don't depend on anyone or anything external to meet your needs.

To practice Aparigraha in everyday life, try:

- Decluttering your house.
- Adopting a minimalist lifestyle.
- Letting go of items, people, places, or habits that no longer serve you.
- Being present in the moment, rather than focusing on the future.
- Practicing and expressing gratitude.
- Practicing forgiveness.
- Carving out time for self-care.
- Genuinely enjoy yourself during your daily yoga flow.
- Practicing your Pranayama exercises and meditation.

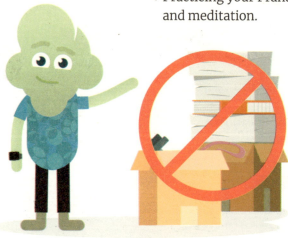

"Yoga is not about self-improvement. It's about self-acceptance."
- Gurmukh Kaur Khalsa

Segment 1: Warm-Up

Full Session Exercise Guide:
habitnest.com/pages/yoga-day-49

1. Thunderbolt Pose w/ Torso Twists
60 sec.

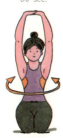

2. Thunderbolt Pose w/ Swinging Arms
30-60 sec.

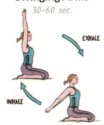

3. Thunderbolt Pose w/ Eagle Arms
30 sec., switch arms & repeat

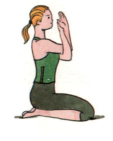

4. Cat-Cow Pose
30-60 sec., alternating

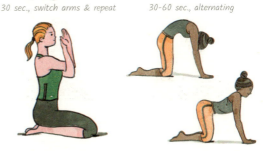

5. Sphinx Pose
60 sec.

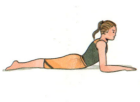

6. Rowing the Boat
30-60 sec.

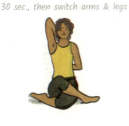

7. Fish Pose Backbend Flow
60 sec.

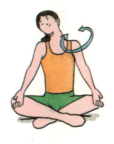

8. Boat Pose Roll-Ups
30-60 sec.

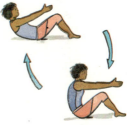

9. Full-Body Stretch to Seated Forward Fold Flow
30-60 sec.

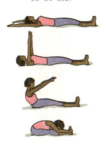

10. Cow Face Pose
30 sec., then switch arms & legs

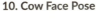

11. Seated Neck Rolls
30 sec. each direction

12. Seated Shoulder Rolls
30 sec. forward & backward

13. Seated Torso Circles
30 sec. each direction

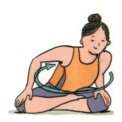

14. Seated Deltoid Stretch
30 sec. per side

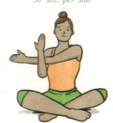

15. Cradle Pose
30 sec. per side

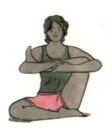

16. Easy Pose Side Bend
30 sec. per side

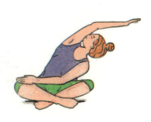

Segment 2: Peak Flow

> Repeat poses 6-12, switching to the opposite side as necessary for asymmetrical poses.

1. Bound Angle Pose
60 sec.

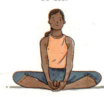

2. Firelog Pose Variation
30 sec. per side

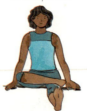

3. Half Cow Face Pose
30 sec. per side

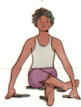

4. Cow Face Pose w/ Eagle Arms
30 sec., then switch arms & legs

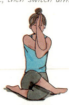

5. Mountain Pose
15 sec.

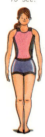

6. Mountain Pose w/ Beginner Eagle Arms
30 sec.

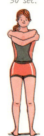

7. Warrior I Pose w/ Eagle Arms
30 sec.

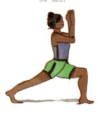

8. Chair Pose w/ Eagle Arms
30 sec.

9. Eagle Pose
30 sec.

10. Chair Pose w/ Cactus Arms
30 sec.

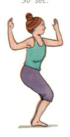

11. Warrior I Pose w/ Cactus Arms
30 sec.

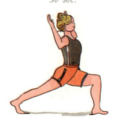

12. Mountain Pose w/ Cactus Arms
30 sec.

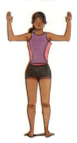

13. Garland Pose
30 sec.

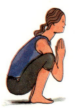

14. Wide Child's Pose
30-60 sec.

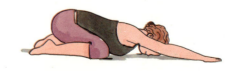

Segment 3: Cool Down

DATE

1. Toe Squat
30-60 sec.

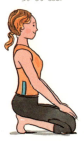

2. Toe Squat w/ Head-to-Knees
30-60 sec.

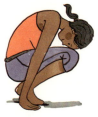

3. Standing Forward Fold
30 sec.

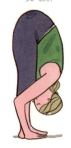

4. Standing Roll-Up Flow
30 sec.

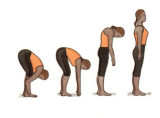

5. Volcano Pose
30 sec.

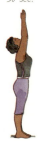

6. Swaying Palm Tree Pose
30 sec. per side

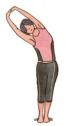

7. Standing Bound Locust Pose
30-60 sec.

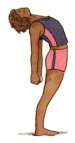

8. Dangling Pose
60 sec.

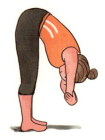

9. Revolved Forward Fold w/ Bent Knee
30 sec. per side

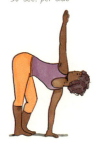

10. Garland Pose
30 sec.

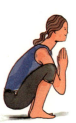

11. Seated Wind Release Pose
60 sec.

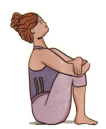

12. Spinal Rock Pose
30-60 sec.

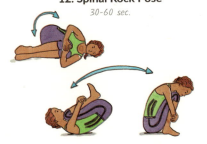

13. Corpse Pose
5 mins.

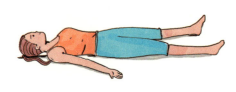

Food for Thought

Niyamas: Ishvara Pranidhana (surrender).

The last of the Niyamas, Ishvara Pranidhana, is translated as 'devotion' or 'surrendering to God.'

Again, this doesn't have to be a specified religion's God or divine being, it could simply be the divinity within yourself that you're seeking to tap into.

In essence, this Niyama is about forming trust, faith, and connection with the universal life force we're all connected to.

This seems easy enough, but surrendering our control isn't always as easy and painless as we think it'll be.

Surrender is often viewed as weak, but in this context, it's a sign of strength and inner peace.

Today, think of an area of your life in which your feel stuck or overwhelmed.

Instead of asking for help from a higher power, ask instead that these feelings will be replaced with peace and understanding.

Instead of fighting against the twists and turns in life, lean into them and open your heart and mind to whatever lessons those twists and turns hold for you.

Surrender the worries you feel, and allow faith to take over.

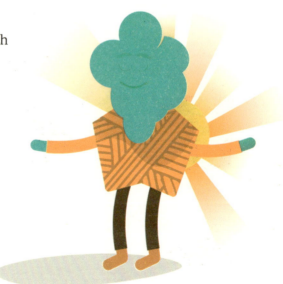

"Letting go is the hardest asana. Tuning in and surrendering the self, body, and soul, to yoga and just being." - Raashi Khanna

Segment 1: Warm-Up

Full Session Exercise Guide:
habitnest.com/pages/yoga-day-50

1. Child's Pose w/ Raised Hips
30-60 sec.

2. Table Top Pose
30 sec.

3. Thread the Needle Pose Flow
60 sec. per side

4. Table Top w/ Leg Extended
30 sec. per side

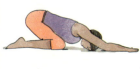
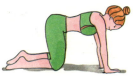
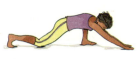
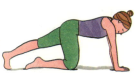

5. Downward Dog to Three-Legged Downward Dog Pose Flow
30 sec. per side

6. Lizard Pose
30-60 sec. per side

7. Lizard Pose w/ Arms Forward
30 sec. per side

8. Sage Twist Pose
30 sec. per side

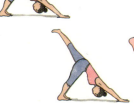
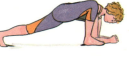
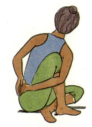

9. Supported Side Plank
30 sec. per side

10. Wild Thing Pose
30 sec. per side

11. Plank Pose
30 sec.

12. Downward Dog to Upward Dog Pose Flow
30 sec.

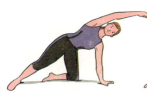

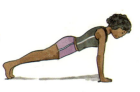

13. Plank Pose w/ Knee to Elbow
30 sec. per side

14. Downward-Facing Dog Pose w/ Hips Side-to-Side
30 sec.

15. Downward Dog to Mountain Pose Flow
30-60 sec.

16. Dangling Intense Leg Stretch Pose
60 sec.

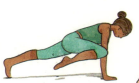
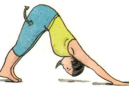
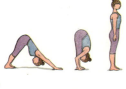
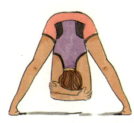

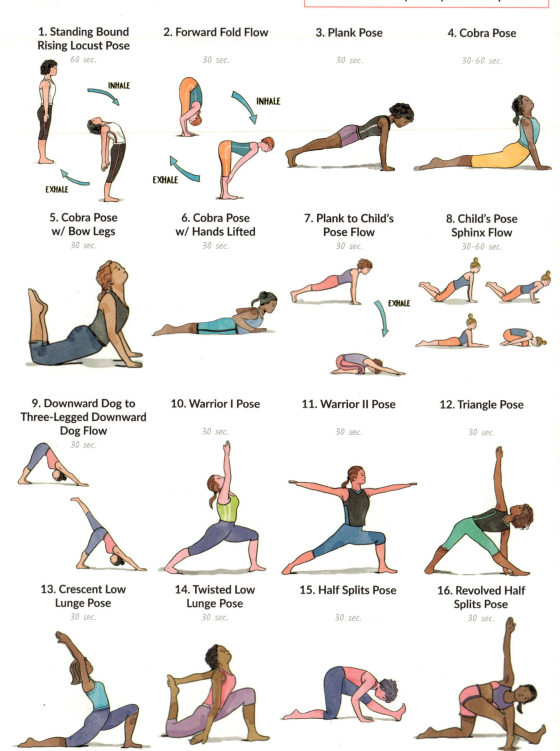

Segment 3: Cool Down

DATE

1. Easy Pose w/ Elbows on Floor
30-60 sec.

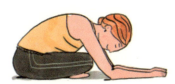

2. Seated Straddle Forward Fold
30-60 sec.

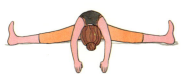

3. Sitting Swan Pose
30 sec. per side

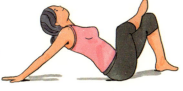

4. Seated Wind Release Pose
30-60 sec.

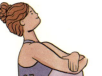

5. Easy Boat Pose
30-60 sec.

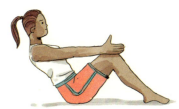

6. Boat Pose B
30 sec.

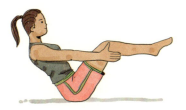

7. Full-Body Stretch Pose
30 sec.

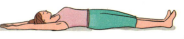

8. Fish Pose
60 sec.

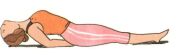

9. Bridge Pose
30-60 sec.

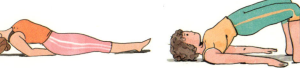

10. Supine Spinal Twist II Pose
30 sec. per side

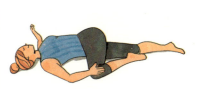

11. Wind Release Pose Breath Flow
30-60 sec.

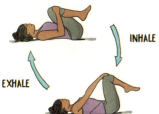

12. Corpse Pose
5 mins.

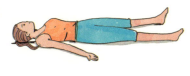

Pro-Tip

Asanas: Preparing your body for more advanced poses.

While advanced yoga poses aren't required, they're a great way to challenge yourself, improve your strength and balance, and deepen your practice – but only with adequate physical and mental preparation!

Be sure to know your limitations, and don't push your body past those limitations.

If you've been sticking to your daily yoga routines (kudos to you!), you've likely already built more strength, flexibility, and mobility, which is helpful for making sure your body is prepared for the challenge.

Some advanced poses, such as headstands or handstands, require you to target and develop specific areas of your body, such as your core, arms, and shoulders. Make sure that you're feeling mentally capable of tackling challenging poses as well.

If you're not quite ready yet, there's no shame in that! Feel free to use modifications and props to make advanced poses accessible and comfortable for your body.

Blocks, bolsters, and straps are all great tools for helping you achieve the poses while also building your way up to being able to perform the poses without props in the future.

Train consistently, listen to your body, and approach each pose mindfully!

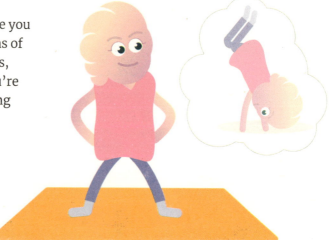

"The study of asana is not about mastering posture. It's about using posture to understand and transform yourself." -B.K.S. Iyengar

Segment 1: Warm-Up

Full Session Exercise Guide:
habitnest.com/pages/yoga-day-51

1. Wrist Flexion/ Extension
30 sec.

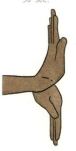

2. Wrist Rotations
30 sec.

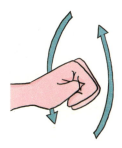

3. Neck Twists
30 sec., alternating sides

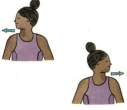

4. Standing Ankle Rotation
30 sec. per side

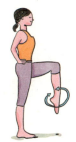

5. Standing Knee Rotation
30-60 sec. per side

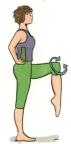

6. Leg Kicks Flow
30 sec. per side

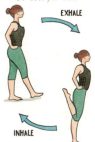

7. Side Lunge Pose w/ Arms Raised
30 sec. per side

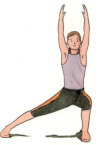

8. Standing Pelvic Circles
30 sec. each direction

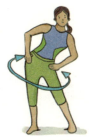

9. Intense Side Stretch
30 sec. per side

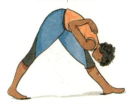

10. Standing Backbend Pose
60 sec.

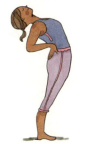

11. Standing Forward Fold Pose
30 sec.

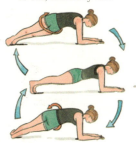

12. Plank Pose w/ Knee-to-Elbow
30 sec. per side

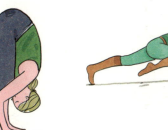

13. Forearm Plank Flow
60 sec.

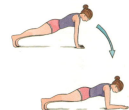

14. Forearm Plank Hip Twists
60 sec., alternating sides

15. Sphinx Pose
60 sec.

16. Sphinx Pose Cat-Cow Flow
60 sec.

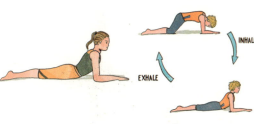

Segment 2: Peak Flow

> Repeat each pose in this segment, switching to the opposite side as necessary for asymmetrical poses.

1. Downward-Facing Dog Pose
30 sec.

2. Crescent Low Lunge Pose
30 sec.

3. Low Lunge Pose
30 sec.

4. Revolved Crescent Low Lunge Pose
30 sec.

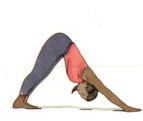
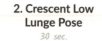
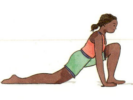
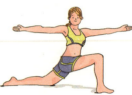

5. Runners Lunge Pose
30 sec.

6. Forward Fold Flow
30 sec.

7. Revolved Forward Fold w/ Bent Knee
30 sec.

8. Mountain Pose
30 sec.

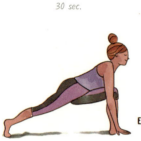
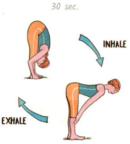
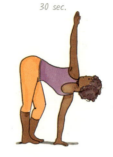
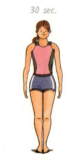

9. Tree Pose
30 sec.

10. Eagle Pose
30 sec.

11. Eagle Pose Crunch
30 sec.

12. Warrior II Pose
30 sec.

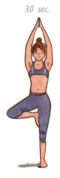
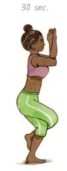
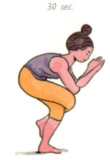
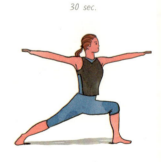

13. Triangle Pose
30 sec.

14. Vinyasa II
60 sec.

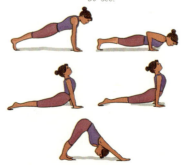

Segment 3: Cool Down

DATE

1. Thunderbolt Pose Salute
60 sec.

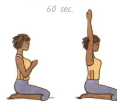

2. Puppy Dog Pose
30-60 sec.

3. Staff Pose
30 sec.

4. Seated Forward Fold Pose
60 sec.

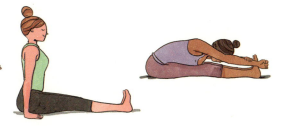

5. Sitting Swan Pose
30 sec. per side

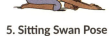

6. Upward Facing Seated Straddle Pose
30-60 sec.

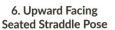

7. Seated Straddle Pose w/ Head-to-Forearms
30-60 sec.

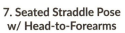

8. Cosmic Egg Pose
30-60 sec.

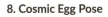

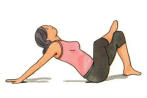
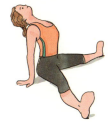
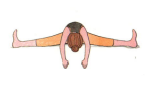
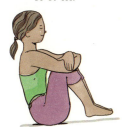

9. Happy Baby Pose
30-60 sec.

10. Reclining Bound Angle Pose
60 sec.

11. Constructive Rest Pose
30-60 sec.

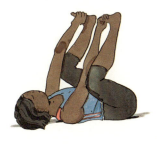
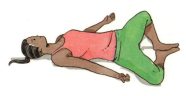
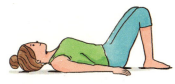

12. Supine Spinal Twist Pose
30 sec. per side

13. Corpse Pose
5 mins.

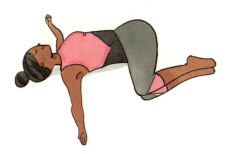
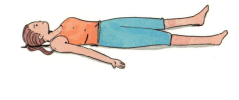

Actionable Challenge

Pratyahara: gratitude.

Gratitude is incredibly helpful for shifting your perspective and learning to genuinely appreciate your life in the present, regardless of what you have or what's going on in your life.

According to research performed by the lead gratitude researcher, Robert Emmons, consistently practicing gratitude is proven to reduce stress, calm the mind, improve focus, and increase happiness!

Today, challenge yourself to practice gratitude in one or more of the following ways:

- Write a **list of 10 things** you're grateful for.
- **Verbally** express genuine gratitude to someone, even if it's just the barista that hands you your morning coffee.
- **Pay it forward** with random acts of kindness.
- Write a **gratitude letter.**
- Call **someone you care about** and thank them for being part of your life.
- Express gratitude to **your body** for getting you to this point and allowing you to experience life.

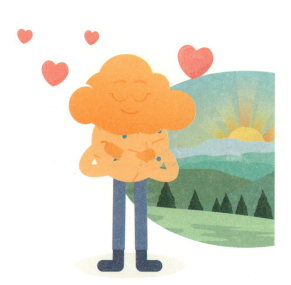

Actionable Challenge Completed: ☐

"The attitude of gratitude is the highest yoga." - Yogi Bhajan

Segment 1: Warm-Up

Full Session Exercise Guide:
habitnest.com/pages/yoga-day-52

1. Revolved Staff Pose Flow
30-60 sec., alternating

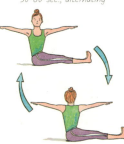

2. Seated Ankle Rotation
30 sec. each direction

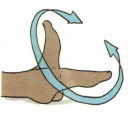

3. Seated Knee Rotation
30 sec. per side

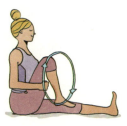

4. Seated Hip Rotation
30 sec. per side

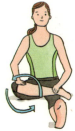

5. Shoulder Socket Rotation
30-60 sec.

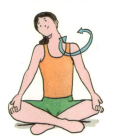

6. Neck Rolls
30 sec. each direction

7. Easy Pose Mudra Flow
30 sec.

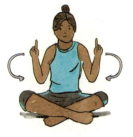

8. Wrist Rolls w/ Hands Clasped
30 sec.

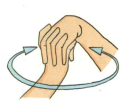

9. Easy Pose Bound Arm Rolls
30 sec. each direction

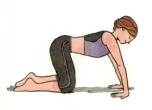

10. Easy Pose w/ Bound Hands
30-60 sec.

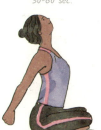

11. Easy Pose Forward Fold
60 sec.

12. Cat-Cow Rib Circles
30-60 sec.

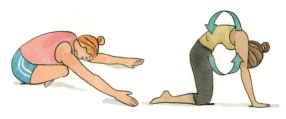

13. Table Top Pose Wrist Stretch
30-60 sec.

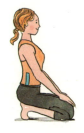

14. Toe Squat
30-60 sec.

15. Thunderbolt Pose Ankle Stretch
30-60 sec.

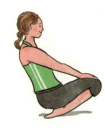

16. Spinal Rock Pose
30-60 sec.

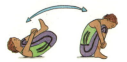

Segment 2: Peak Flow

1. Revolved Figure Four Pose
30-60 sec. per side

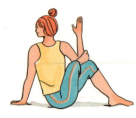

2. Sitting Swan Pose
30 sec. per side

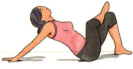

3. Reverse Table Top Pose
30-60 sec.

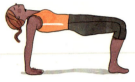

4. One-Legged Reverse Table Top Pose
30 sec. per side

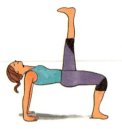

5. Upward Plank Pose
30-60 sec.

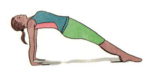

6. Boat Pose
30-60 sec.

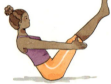

7. Reclined Eagle Crunches
60 sec.

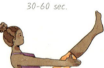

8. Wind Release to Mountain Pose Flow
30-60 sec.

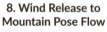
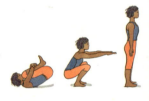

9. Chair Pose
30 sec.

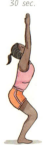

10. Standing Forward Fold Pose
60 sec.

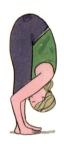

11. Plank to Downward Dog Pose Flow
30 sec.

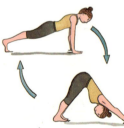
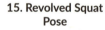

12. Puppy Dog Pose
30-60 sec.

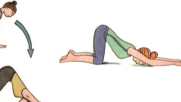

13. Revolved Downward-Facing Dog Pose
30 sec. per side

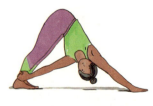

14. Garland Pose
30 sec.

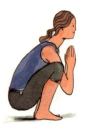

15. Revolved Squat Pose
30 sec. per side

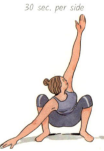

16. Wide Child's Pose
30-60 sec.

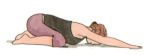

Segment 3: Cool Down

DATE

1. Bound Angle Pose
60 sec.

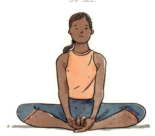

2. Seated Star Pose
60 sec.

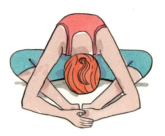

3. Half Lord of the Fishes Pose
30 sec. per side

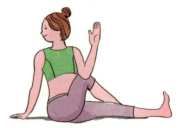

4. Sitting Swan Pose
30 sec. per side

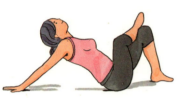

5. Happy Baby Pose
30-60 sec.

6. Supine Spinal Twist II Pose
30 sec. per side

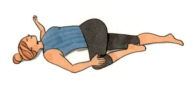

7. Half Plow Pose
30-60 sec.

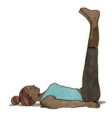

8. Fish Pose
60 sec.

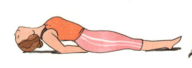

9. Reclining Bound Angle
30-60 sec.

10. Full-Body Stretch Pose
30 sec.

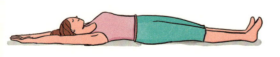

11. Corpse Pose
5 mins.

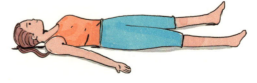

Actionable Challenge

Dharana: mantras & chants.

In Yoga, sounds in the form of spoken mantras and chants can enhance and complement our daily practice.

They awaken, control, and direct our energy in order to deepen our mind-body connection and shift our consciousness in a meditative way.

Mantra translates roughly to "vehicle of the mind", which is because it directs and drives our bodily energies.

The mantras you choose for yourself can be anything that you find helpful, such as:

- "I am confident in my abilities."
- "I have an abundance of energy and strength."
- "I am powerful and in control of my life."

Chants, on the other hand, are the meditative sounds we make. You may have noticed that each Chakra has a corresponding sound, such as Om, Aum, Lam, Yam, etc.

These sounds are designed to positively alter your consciousness and cultivate a meditative state that grounds us and connects us to the divine within us.

Before you start your practice today, choose a mantra and the sound for whichever Chakra you need to balance.

Meditating on your mantra will help you create a sense of peace and ambiance, while the sound will help you tap into and balance your Chakras.

When you notice your mind drifting away from your intended focus, simply return to your mantra and chant to get your brain back in the game.

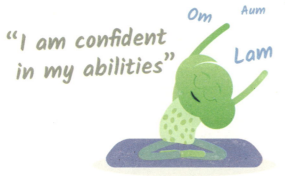

Actionable Challenge Completed: ☐

"Meditation can help us embrace our worries, our fear, our anger; and that is very healing. We let our own natural capacity of healing do the work." - Thich Nhat Hahn

Segment 1: Warm-Up

Full Session Exercise Guide:
habitnest.com/pages/yoga-day-53

1. Supine Arm Sweep I
30-60 sec.

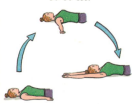

2. Supine Arm Sweep II
30-60 sec.

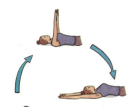

3. Half Wind Release Pose
30 sec. per side

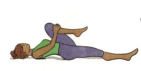

4. Dead Bug Core Exercise II
1-2 mins., alternating

5. Staff Pose
30 sec.

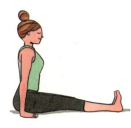

6. Seated Forward Fold Pose
60 sec.

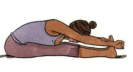

7. Staff Pose Knee Stretches
30 sec. per side

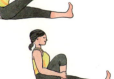

8. Half Lord of the Fishes Pose
30 sec. per side

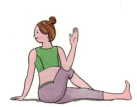

9. Cradle Pose
30 sec. per side

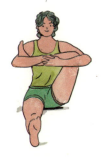

10. Seated Neck Rolls
30 sec. each direction

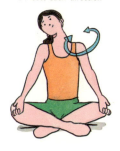

11. Wrist Rolls w/ Clasped Hands
30 sec.

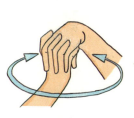

12. Cat-Cow Pose
30-60 sec., alternating

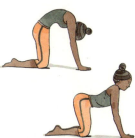

13. Balancing Table Top Knee-to-Nose Crunches
30 sec. per side

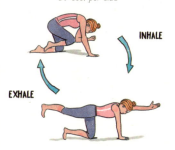

14. Child's Pose
30-60 sec.

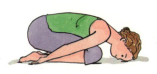

15. Simple Grounded Shakti Flow
1-2 mins.

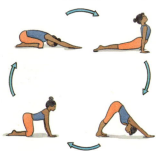

Segment 2: Peak Flow

> Repeat poses 1-14, switching to the opposite side as necessary for asymmetrical poses.

1. Downward-Facing Dog Pose
30 sec.

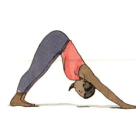

2. Crescent Low Lunge Pose
30 sec.

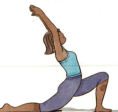

3. Low Lunge Pose
30 sec.

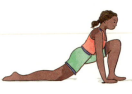

4. Revolved Crescent Low Lunge Pose
30 sec.

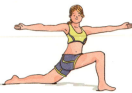

5. Runners Lunge Pose
30 sec.

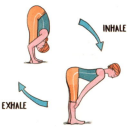

6. Forward Fold Flow
30 sec.

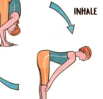

7. Revolved Forward Fold w/ Bent Knee
30 sec.

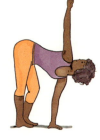

8. Mountain Pose
30 sec.

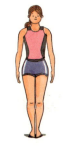

9. Tree Pose
30 sec.

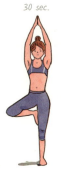

10. Eagle Pose
30 sec.

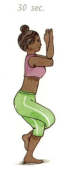

11. Eagle Pose Crunch
30 sec.

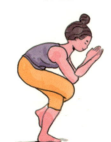

12. Warrior II Pose
30 sec.

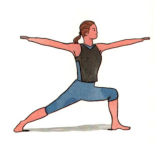

13. Triangle Pose
30 sec.

14. Vinyasa II
60 sec.

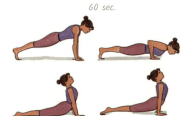

Segment 3: Cool Down

DATE

1. Downward-Facing Dog Pose
30 sec.

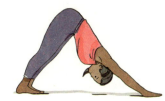

2. Pigeon Pose
30 sec. per side

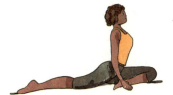

3. Sleeping Swan Pose
30-60 sec. per side

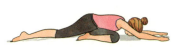

4. Revolved Pigeon Pose
30 sec. per side

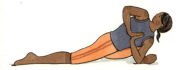

5. Head-to-Knee Pose
30 sec. per side

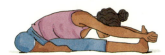

6. Revolved Head-to-Knee Pose
30 sec. per side

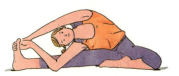

7. Bridge Pose
30-60 sec.

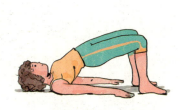

8. One-Legged Bridge Pose
30 sec. per side

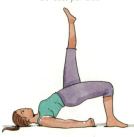

9. Happy Baby Pose
30-60 sec.

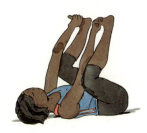

10. Supine Spinal Twist II Pose
30 sec. per side

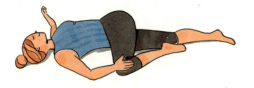

11. Corpse Pose
5 mins.

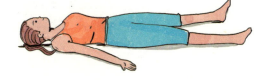

Favorite Resources

Dhyana: check out the *Yoga by Nature* podcast.

Need a yoga flow or meditation on the go? The 'Yoga by Nature' podcast is a great option! This podcast is chock full of audio-guided yoga flows, meditation, and even Yoga Nidra.

Yoga Nidra is essentially a yogic sleep that promotes deep whole-body relaxation.

The podcasts range anywhere from 10-90 minutes with over 40 guided Hatha flows that help you to build strength, take care of your joints, and improve your flexibility and mobility.

Their options are suitable for beginners and target a range of different focuses. There's definitely something for everyone on the Yoga by Nature podcast!

You can find this podcast by searching for it online, or on Apple Podcasts.

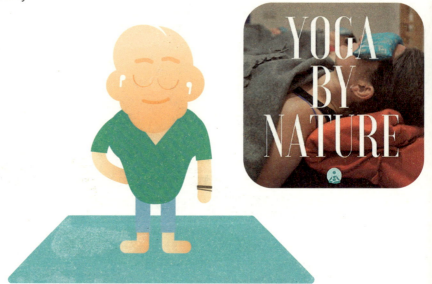

"The gift of learning to meditate is the greatest gift you can give yourself in this lifetime." - Sogyal Rinpoche

Segment 1: Warm-Up

Full Session Exercise Guide:
habitnest.com/pages/yoga-day-54

1. Corpse Pose
60 sec.

2. Banana Pose
30 sec. per side

3. Wind Release Pose
60 sec.

4. Circle of Joy
60 sec.

5. Cat-Cow Pose
30-60 sec., alternating

6. Tiger Pose
30 sec. per side

7. Child's Pose w/ Arms to One Side
30 sec per side.

8. Child's Pose Sun Salutation
1-2 mins.

9. Thunderbolt Pose w/ Swinging Arms
30 sec.

10. Shoulder Socket Rotations
30-60 sec.

11. Cow Face Arms
30 sec. per side

12. Standing Forward Fold Pose
30 sec.

13. Standing Roll-Up Flow
30-60 sec.

14. Standing Circle of Joy
60 sec.

15. Breath of Joy
60-90 sec.

Segment 2: Peak Flow

> Repeat poses 1-12, switching to the opposite side as necessary for asymmetrical poses.

1. Palm Tree Pose w/ Bound Elbows
30 sec.

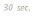

2. Mountain Pose Tiptoes Flow
30 sec.

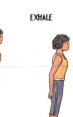

3. Five-Pointed Star Pose
30 sec.

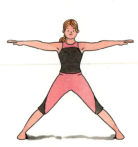

4. Revolved Wide-Legged Forward Fold Pose
30 sec.

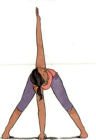

5. Goddess Pose
30-45 sec.

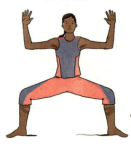

6. Revolved Side Angle Pose
30 sec.

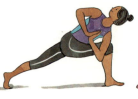

7. Revolved Side Angle Pose w/ Hand to Floor
30 sec.

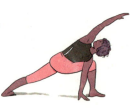

8. Half Moon Pose
30 sec.

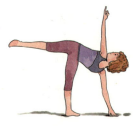

9. Warrior III Pose
30 sec.

10. Runners Lunge Pose
30 sec.

11. Revolved Lunge Pose
30 sec.

12. Goddess Pose w/ Eagle Arms
30 sec.

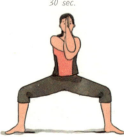

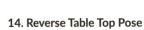

13. Boat Pose
30-60 sec.

14. Reverse Table Top Pose
30 sec.

15. Bridge Pose
30-60 sec.

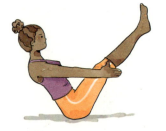
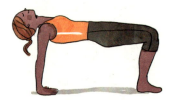
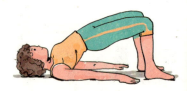

Segment 3: Cool Down

DATE

1. Rolling Happy Baby Variation Flow
60 sec.

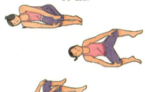

2. Bound Reclined Easy Pose
30-60 sec.

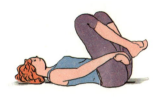

3. Half Plow Pose
30-60 sec.

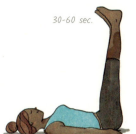

4. Supine Spinal Twist Pose
30 sec. per side

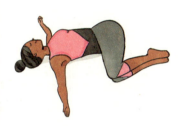

5. Seated Forward Fold Pose
60 sec.

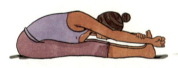

6. Half Happy Baby Pose
30 sec. per side

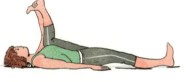

7. Sitting Swan Pose
30 sec. per side

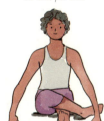

8. Half Cow Face Pose
30 sec. per side

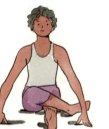

9. Half Cow Face Pose w/ Forward Fold
30 sec. per side

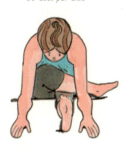

10. Full-Body Stretch Pose
30 sec.

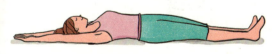

11. Corpse Pose
5 mins.

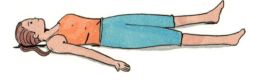

Food for Thought

Chakras: Throat Chakra (Vishuddha)

The Throat Chakra, located in the center of your throat, is the energetic command center for communication. It focuses both on speaking up for yourself, and on being heard by others.

A balanced Throat Chakra helps you to communicate smoothly with others, and tying this Chakra to your Sacral Chakra allows optimal creativity flow.

It's associated with these characteristics:

- **Color** - Blue
- **Element** - Ether/Space
- **Sound** - Ham

An imbalanced Throat Chakra can make you feel more fearful of speaking to others, lead you to stay quiet, and prevents you from feeling able to express yourself openly.

In contrast, an overactive Throat Chakra might lead you to be overly talkative or rambling.

To bring your Throat Chakra back to working order, try:

- Practicing your Pranayama exercises.
- Drinking warm tea or herbal drinks with honey to keep your throat in tip-top shape.
- Practicing asanas that involve stretching the neck.
- Singing, chanting, or humming to create soothing vibrations in the throat.
- Fearlessly being your genuine, authentic self.

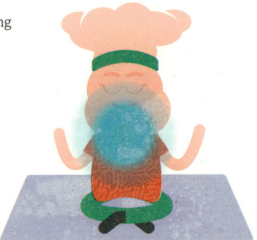

"True success is achieved by stretching oneself, learning to feel comfortable being uncomfortable." - Ken Poirot

Segment 1: Warm-Up

Full Session Exercise Guide:
habitnest.com/pages/yoga-day-55

1. Child's Pose w/ Raised Hips
30-60 sec.

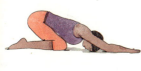

2. Table Top Pose
30 sec.

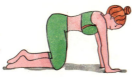

3. Thread the Needle Pose Flow
30 sec. per side

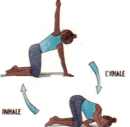

4. Table Top w/ Leg Extended
30 sec. per side

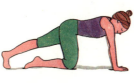

5. Downward Dog to Three-Legged Downward Dog Pose Flow
30 sec.

6. Lizard Pose
30-60 sec. per side

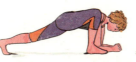

7. Lizard Pose w/ Arms Forward
30 sec.

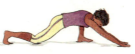

8. Sage Twist Pose
30 sec.

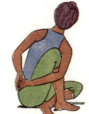

9. Supported Side Plank
30 sec.

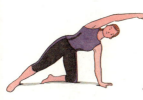

10. Wild Thing Pose
30 sec.

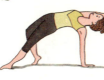

11. Plank Pose
30 sec.

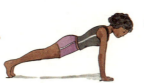

12. Downward Dog to Upward Dog Pose Flow
30 sec.

13. Plank Pose w/ Knee to Elbow
30 sec. per side

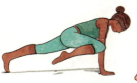

14. Downward-Facing Dog Pose w/ Hips Side-to-Side
30-60 sec.

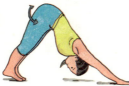

15. Downward Dog to Mountain Pose Flow
30-60 sec.

16. Dangling Intense Leg Stretch Pose
60 sec.

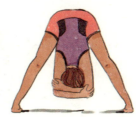

Repeat poses 5-11, switching to the opposite side as necessary for asymmetrical poses.

Segment 2: Peak Flow

> Repeat poses 1-12, switching to the opposite side as necessary for asymmetrical poses.

1. Downward Dog to Three-Legged Downward Dog Pose Flow
30-60 sec.

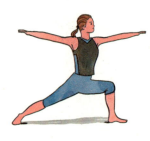

2. Fallen Triangle Pose
30 sec.

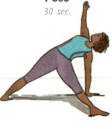

3. Runner's Lunge Pose
30 sec.

4. Triangle Pose Side Stretch
30 sec.

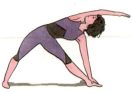

5. Warrior II Pose
30 sec.

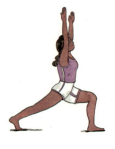

6. Downward Dog to Three-Legged Downward Dog Pose Flow
30 sec.

7. Low Lunge Pose
30 sec.

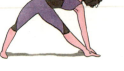

8. Low Lunge w/ Tricep Stretch
30 sec.

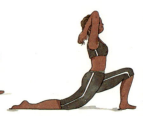

9. High Lunge Pose
30 sec.

10. Revolved High Lunge Pose
30 sec.

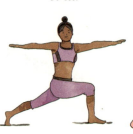

11. Side Lunge Pose
30 sec.

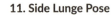

12. Wide-Legged Lateral Squat
30 sec.

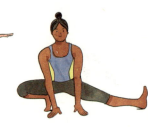

13. Plank Pose
30 sec.

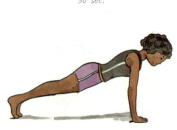

14. Vinyasa II
60 sec.

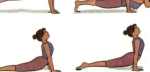

15. Thunderbolt Pose
30-60 sec.

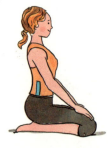

Segment 3: Cool Down

DATE

1. Thunderbolt Pose w/ Cat-Cow
30 sec.

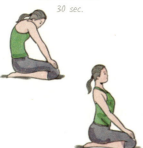

2. Revolved Thunderbolt Pose
30 sec. per side

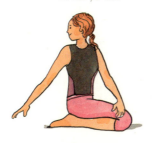

3. Thunderbolt Pose Salute
60 sec.

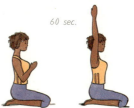

4. Puppy Dog Pose
30-60 sec.

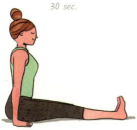

5. Resting Half Frog Pose
30 sec. per side

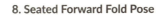

6. Seated Wind Release Pose
30-60 sec.

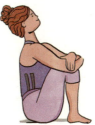

7. Staff Pose
30 sec.

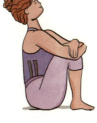

8. Seated Forward Fold Pose
60 sec.

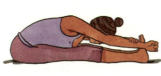

9. Sitting Swan Pose
30 sec. per side

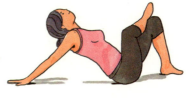

10. Happy Baby Pose
30-60 sec.

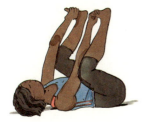

11. Reclining Bound Angle Pose
30-60 sec.

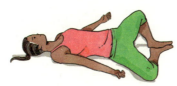

12. Corpse Pose
5 mins.

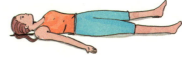

Food for Thought

Koshas: Anandamaya.

The last and most all-encompassing layer of our existence is the Anandamaya Kosha, which translates to our 'bliss sheath.'

This sheath corresponds to the element of ether/space, and it focuses not on feeling ecstatic joy, but on creating an unshakeable, steady-state of being regardless of the circumstances.

Realize that you are whole, regardless of outcomes and external obstacles.

Unlike the previous four Koshas, this Kosha isn't something you achieve or balance.

It's not even something that can be accurately pinned down, defined, or contemplated. It is something you continuously experience and work toward.

Seek the steady state of bliss that you would find in a child who is fully immersed in the present moment, and work to cultivate that sense of immersion and experience. Focus on being, rather than doing.

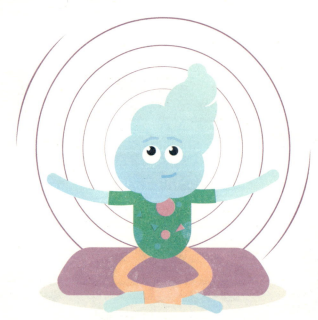

"Peace comes from within. Do not seek it without." - Gautama Buddha

Segment 1: Warm-Up

Full Session Exercise Guide:
habitnest.com/pages/yoga-day-56

1. Alternate Nostril Breathing
2-4 mins.

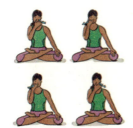

2. Alternating Shoulder Shrugs
30 sec.

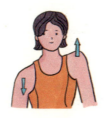

3. Alternating Elbow Flapping
30 sec.

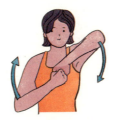

4. Deltoid Stretch
30 sec. per side

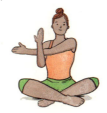

5. Wrist Flexion/ Extension
30 sec.

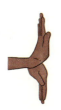

6. Wrist Rotations
30 sec.

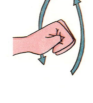

7. Seated Torso Circles
30 sec. each direction

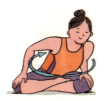

8. Easy Pose Side Bend
30 sec. per side

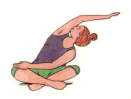

9. Revolved Easy Pose Salute Flow
30-60 sec., alternating sides

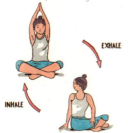

10. Seated Knee Rotations
30 sec. per side

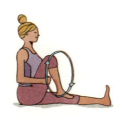

11. Cradle Pose
30 sec. per side

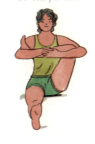

12. Staff Pose w/ Alternating Knee & Hand Lifts
30 sec.

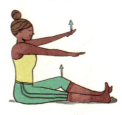

13. Boat to Half Boat Pose Flow
30-60 sec.

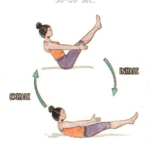

14. Half Plow Rollover Flow
30-60 sec.

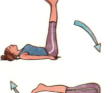

15. Spinal Rock Pose
60 sec.

16. Wind Release to Mountain Pose Flow
30-60 sec.

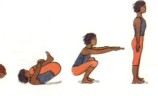

Segment 2: Peak Flow

> Repeat poses 1-12, switching to the opposite side as necessary for asymmetrical poses.

1. Chair Pose
30 sec.

2. Straight-Legged Warrior I Salute Flow
30 sec.

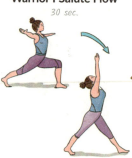

3. Warrior II Intense Leg Stretch Flow
60 sec.

4. Revolved Wide-Legged Forward Fold Pose
30-60 sec.

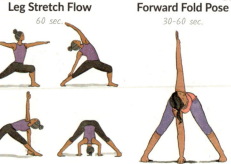

5. Goddess Pose
30-45 sec.

6. Warrior II Pose
30 sec.

7. Reverse Warrior Pose
30 sec.

8. Warrior III Pose
30 sec.

9. Sugarcane Pose
30 sec.

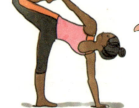

10. Half Moon Pose
30 sec.

11. Dancer Pose
30 sec.

12. Standing Forward Fold Pose
30 sec.

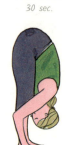

13. Garland Pose
30 sec.

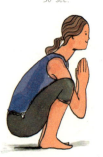

14. Bound Angle Pose
60 sec.

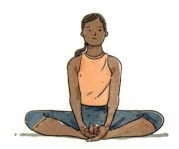

Segment 3: Cool Down

DATE

1. Easy Pose w/ Elbows on Floor
30-60 sec.

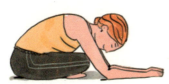

2. Seated Straddle Forward Fold
30-60 sec.

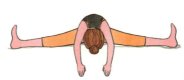

3. Sitting Swan Pose
30 sec. per side

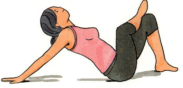

4. Seated Wind Release Pose
30-60 sec.

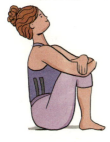

5. Easy Boat Pose
30-60 sec.

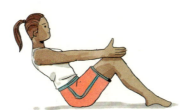

6. Boat Pose B
30 sec.

7. Full-Body Stretch Pose
30 sec.

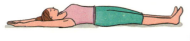

8. Fish Pose
60 sec.

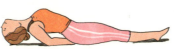

9. Bridge Pose
30-60 sec.

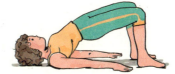

10. Supine Spinal Twist II Pose
30 sec. per side

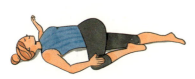

11. Wind Release Pose Breath Flow
30-60 sec.

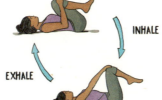

12. Corpse Pose
5 mins.

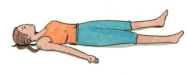

Pro-Tip

Try a yoga swing.

Even as early as 3,000 B.C., rope devices were used as rudimentary yoga swings in order to provide support and assistance in your asana practice.

It can decompress the joints and spine (especially if you do any inversion poses), prevent injuries, and allow for more dynamic asana practice.

Consider giving a yoga swing a try! Some of the most popular yoga swing brands on the market include Gravatonics, Omni, and YOGABODY.

Before using a yoga swing, make sure you:

- You clear it with your doctor first, especially if you have any medical conditions, past surgeries, or recent injuries.

- Don't use the swing on a full stomach. Give your meal at least 2-3 hours to settle and start digesting.

- Read over the user manual and ensure that everything is safely mounted

- Wear clothes that cover your skin to prevent friction burns or rashes, and don't wear any loose clothing items, accessories, or embellishments that could get tangled up in the swing.

- Take it slow and easy!

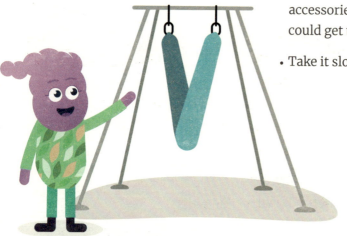

"Yoga isn't just repetition of a few postures, it is more about the exploration and discovery of the subtle energies of life." - Amit Ray

Segment 1: Warm-Up

Full Session Exercise Guide:
habitnest.com/pages/yoga-day-57

1. Bound Angle Pose
60 sec.

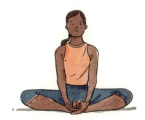

2. Cradle Pose
30 sec. per side

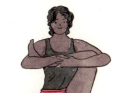

3. Head-to-Knee Pose
30 sec. per side

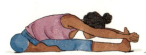

4. Revolved Head-to-Knee Pose
30 sec. per side

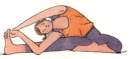

5. Crocodile Pose
30 sec.

6. Locust Pose
30-60 sec.

7. Dolphin Pose
60 sec.

8. Three-Legged Downward-Facing Dog Pose
30 sec.

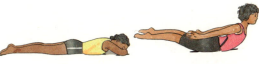

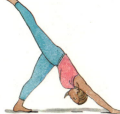

9. Lizard Pose
30-60 sec.

10. Triangle Pose w/ Bent Knee
30 sec.

11. Standing Forward Fold Pose
30 sec.

12. Dangling Pose
30 sec.

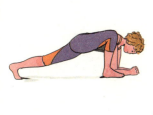
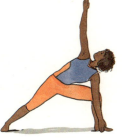
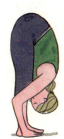
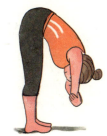

13. Chair Pose
30 sec.

14. Standing Backbend Pose
30-60 sec.

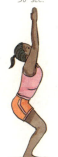
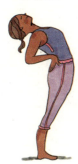

> Repeat poses 8-10, switching to the opposite side as necessary for asymmetrical poses.

Segment 2: Peak Flow

> Repeat poses 1-12, switching to the opposite side as necessary for asymmetrical poses.

1. Palm Tree Pose w/ Bound Elbows
30 sec.

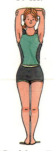

2. Mountain Pose Tiptoes Flow
30 sec.

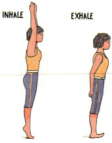

3. Five-Pointed Star Pose
30 sec.

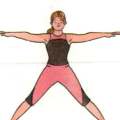

4. Revolved Wide-Legged Forward Fold Pose
30 sec.

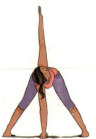

5. Goddess Pose
30-45 sec.

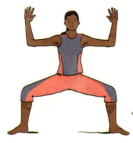

6. Revolved Side Angle Pose
30 sec.

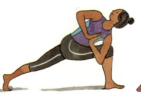

7. Revolved Side Angle Pose w/ Hand to Floor
30 sec.

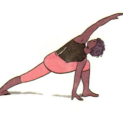

8. Half Moon Pose
30 sec.

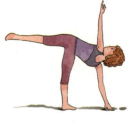

9. Warrior III Pose
30 sec.

10. Runners Lunge Pose
30 sec.

11. Revolved Lunge Pose
30 sec.

12. Goddess Pose w/ Eagle Arms
30 sec.

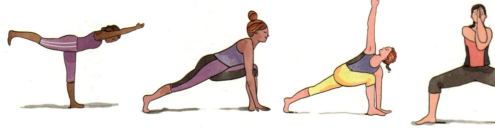
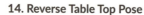
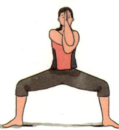

13. Boat Pose
30-60 sec.

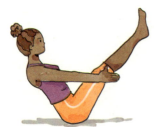

14. Reverse Table Top Pose
30 sec.

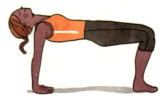

15. Bridge Pose
30-60 sec.

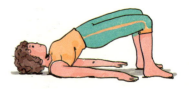

Segment 3: Cool Down

DATE

1. Wind Release Pose
60 sec.

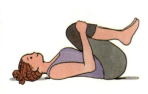

2. Happy Baby Pose
30-60 sec.

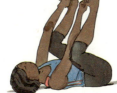

3. Supine Spinal Twist II Pose
30-60 sec. per side

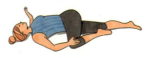

4. Fish Pose
60 sec.

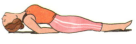

5. Full-Body Stretch Pose
30-60 sec.

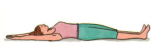

6. Half Plow Pose
30-60 sec.

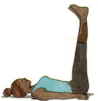

7. Sage Marichi Pose C
30 sec. per side

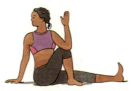

8. Sitting Swan Pose
30 sec. per side

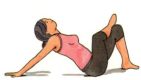

9. Upward-Facing Seated Straddle Pose
30-60 sec.

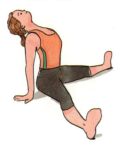

10. Seated Straddle Forward Fold Pose
30-60 sec.

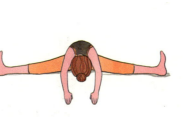

11. Staff Pose
30 sec.

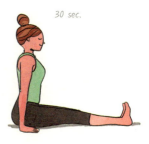

12. Seated Forward Fold Pose
60 sec.

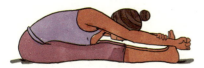

13. Corpse Pose
5 mins.

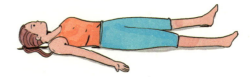

Favorite Resources

Pranayama: *The Breathing Book* **by Donna Farhi.**

Looking to expand your breath control and learn even more breathing techniques? Look no further than *The Breathing Book: Good Health and Vitality Through Essential Breath Work* by Donna Farhi.

This book contains an in-depth program that helps you target your specific breathwork needs, learn to cope with stress, and even improve your physical health, all of which is presented by an experienced and knowledgeable yoga instructor.

It provides tons of illustrations as well, helping to make the exercises easier to understand.

You can find Donna's book by searching for it on Google or Amazon, so check it out and keep up the important Pranayama work!

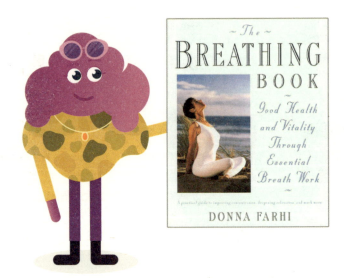

"Spiritual awareness must be brought into our daily life if we are to become receptive to the radiance of that Consciousness that is pulsing with divine vibrations."
- Gurmukh Kaur Khalsa

Segment 1: Warm-Up

Full Session Exercise Guide:
habitnest.com/pages/yoga-day-58

1. Child's Pose w/ Raised Hips
30-60 sec.

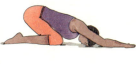

2. Table Top Pose
30 sec.

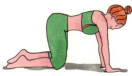

3. Thread the Needle Pose Flow
30 sec. per side

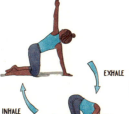

4. Table Top w/ Leg Extended
30 sec. per side

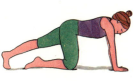

5. Downward Dog to Three-Legged Downward Dog Pose Flow
30 sec.

6. Lizard Pose
30-60 sec. per side

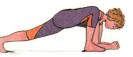

7. Lizard Pose w/ Arms Forward
30 sec.

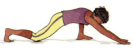

8. Sage Twist Pose
30 sec.

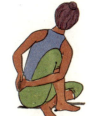

9. Supported Side Plank
30 sec.

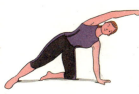

10. Wild Thing Pose
30 sec.

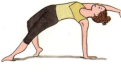

11. Plank Pose
30 sec.

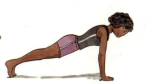

12. Downward Dog to Upward Dog Pose Flow
30 sec.

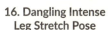

13. Plank Pose w/ Knee to Elbow
30 sec. per side

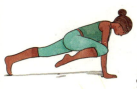

14. Downward-Facing Dog Pose w/ Hips Side-to-Side
30-60 sec.

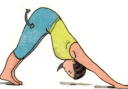

15. Downward Dog to Mountain Pose Flow
30-60 sec.

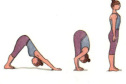

16. Dangling Intense Leg Stretch Pose
60 sec.

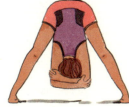

Repeat poses 5-11, switching to the opposite side as necessary for asymmetrical poses.

Segment 2: Peak Flow

> Repeat poses 1-8, switching to the opposite side as necessary for asymmetrical poses.

1. Standing Wind Release Pose
30 sec.

2. Tree Pose
30 sec.

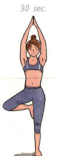

3. Revolved Hand-to-Big-Toe Pose
30 sec.

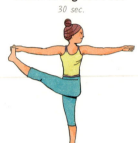

4. Revolved Chair Pose
30 sec.

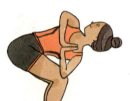

5. High Lunge w/ Arms Extended
30 sec.

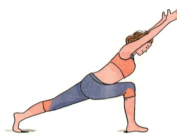

6. Easy Revolved Side Angle Pose
30 sec.

7. Revolved Side Angle Pose
30 sec.

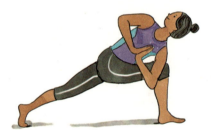

8. Downward Dog Vinyasa Flow
30-60 sec.

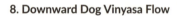
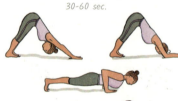
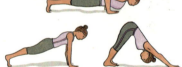

9. Four-Limbed Staff to Plank Push-Up
30-60 sec.

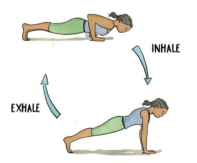

10. Child's Pose
30-60 sec.

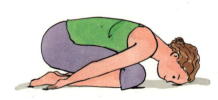

Segment 3: Cool Down

DATE

1. Child's Pose w/ Reverse Prayer
30-60 sec.

2. Table Top Pose
30 sec.

3. Thread the Needle Pose
30-60 sec. per side

4. Staff Pose
30-60 sec.

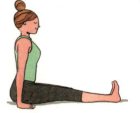
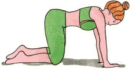
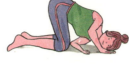

5. Sage Marichi Pose C
30 sec. per side

6. Seated Forward Fold
60 sec.

7. Bound Angle Pose
60 sec.

8. Seated Star Pose
60 sec.

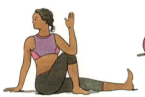
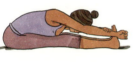
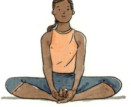
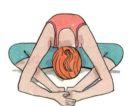

9. Wind Release Pose
60 sec.

10. Half Plow Pose
30-60 sec.

11. Bridge Pose
30-60 sec.

12. Supine Spinal Twist II Pose
30 sec. per side

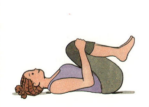
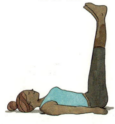
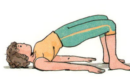
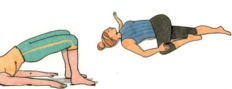

13. Reclining Bound Angle Pose
30-60 sec.

14. Corpse Pose
5 mins.

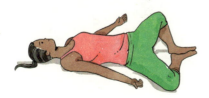
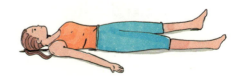

Pro-Tip

Pratyahara: cultivate joy & humor in your practice.

While traditional forms of yoga have plenty of proven health benefits, you can take those benefits up a notch just by practicing laughing yoga.

Laughter Yoga was started by an Indian doctor who was often known as the "Guru of giggling" in 1995 and spread much like contagious laughter.

There's no need to follow a specific flow, just keep your mood light, smile, and laugh throughout your flow.

Laughter is said to be effective against depression, anxiety, and stress, and even to boost your immune system!

Make it a point today to turn your serious energy into "funergy." Be light and playful with yourself, and just allow an abundance of joy and happiness to flow through you.

Yoga requires us to spend so much time being serious about our mind, body, and soul, but that doesn't mean you can't have some fun and let go of self-consciousness!

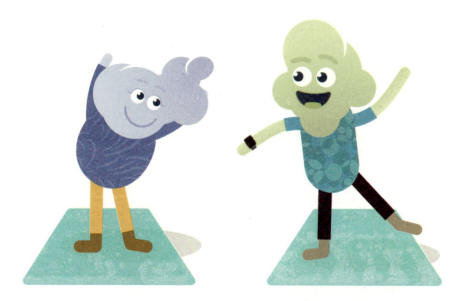

"It is only when the mind is free from the old that it meets everything anew, and in that there is joy." - Jiddu Krishnamurti

Segment 1: Warm-Up

Full Session Exercise Guide:
habitnest.com/pages/yoga-day-59

1. Seated Neck Rolls
30 sec. each direction

2. Easy Pose Mudra Flow
30 sec.

3. Seated Shoulder Rolls
30 sec. forward & backward

4. Cactus Arms Shoulder Movements
60 sec., alternating

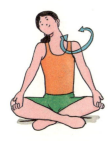

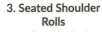
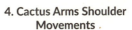

5. Deltoid Stretch
30 sec. per side

6. Side-to-Side Neck Stretch
30 sec. per side

7. Easy Pose Side Bend
30 sec. per side

8. Revolved Easy Pose Salute Flow
30-60 sec., alternating sides

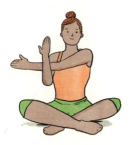

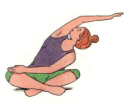

9. Seated Cat-Cow Pose
30-60 sec., alternating

10. Staff Pose
30 sec.

11. Seated Side Straddle Pose
30 sec. per side

12. Upward-Facing Seated Straddle w/ Toe Grab
30-60 sec.

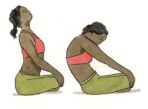
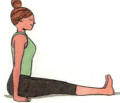
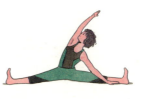
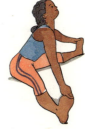

13. Seated Forward Fold Pose
60 sec.

14. Supine Spinal Twist Pose
30 sec. per side

15. Side Reclining Scissors Flow
30-60 sec. per side

16. Side Reclining Leg Lift
30-60 sec. per side

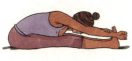
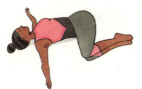
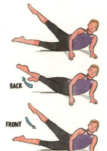
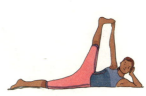

Segment 2: Peak Flow

> Repeat poses 1-12, switching to the opposite side as necessary for asymmetrical poses.

1. Palm Tree Pose w/ Bound Elbows
30 sec.

2. Mountain Pose Tiptoes Flow
30 sec.

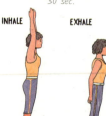

3. Five-Pointed Star Pose
30 sec.

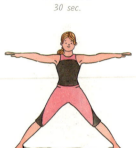

4. Revolved Wide-Legged Forward Fold Pose
30 sec.

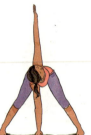

5. Goddess Pose
30-45 sec.

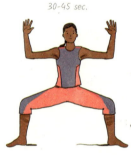

6. Revolved Side Angle Pose
30 sec.

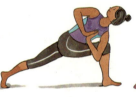

7. Revolved Side Angle Pose w/ Hand to Floor
30 sec.

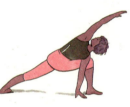

8. Half Moon Pose
30 sec.

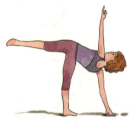

9. Warrior III Pose
30 sec.

10. Runners Lunge Pose
30 sec.

11. Revolved Lunge Pose
30 sec.

12. Goddess Pose w/ Eagle Arms
30-60 sec.

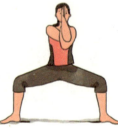

13. Boat Pose
30-60 sec.

14. Reverse Table Top Pose
30 sec.

15. Bridge Pose
30-60 sec.

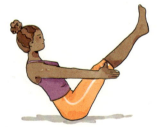
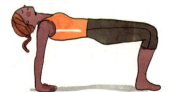
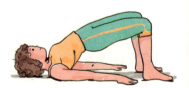

Segment 3: Cool Down

DATE

1. Fish Pose
60 sec.

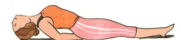

2. Full-Body Stretch Pose
60 sec.

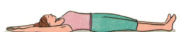

3. Half Wind Release Pose
30 sec. per side

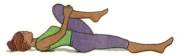

4. Wind Release Pose
60 sec.

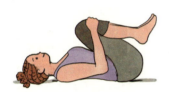

5. Scorpion Twist Pose
30 sec. per side

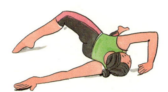

6. Supine Butterfly Pose Wings
30-60 sec.

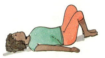
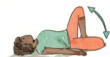

7. Supine Windshield Wipers
30 sec. per side

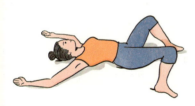

8. Reverse Pigeon Pose
30 sec. per side

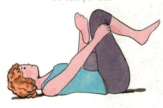

9. Reclined Half Cow Face Pose
30-60 sec. per side

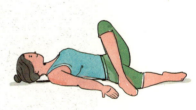

10. Reclined Cow Face Pose
30 sec., then reverse legs & repeat

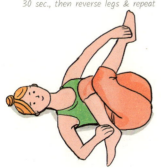

11. Corpse Pose
5 mins.

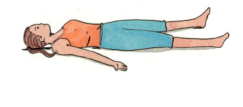

Favorite Resources

Dharana: *The Heart of Yoga* **by T.K.V. Desikachar.**

If you have found value and purpose in developing your practice, don't stop now!

Using a step-by-step process based on the teachings of one of the greatest and most influential Yogis to have developed the practice of yoga - Krishnamacharya.

The program adapts to your needs to maximize the therapeutic value of your practice.

T.K.V. Desikachar, the son of Krishnamacharya, wrote this book to encompass the entirety of his father's teachings, as well as some of his own approaches, in a way that could be easily customized to fit the reader's health, career, age, and complete lifestyle.

You're nearing the end of your 66-day journey, and if you're not ready to stop developing your yoga practice, *"The Heart of Yoga: Developing a Personal Practice"* by T.K.V. Desikachar is the perfect book for you! You can find it by searching for it on Google or Amazon.

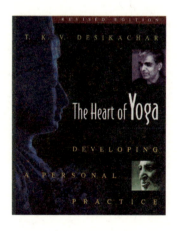
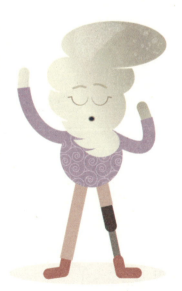

"The success of yoga does not lie in the ability to perform postures, but in how it positively changes the way we live our life and our relationships."- T.K.V. Desikachar

Segment 1: Warm-Up

Full Session Exercise Guide:
habitnest.com/pages/yoga-day-60

1. Alternate Nostril Breathing
2-4 mins.

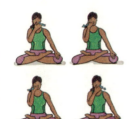

2. Alternating Shoulder Shrugs
30 sec.

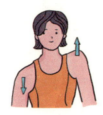

3. Alternating Elbow Flapping
30 sec.

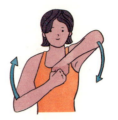

4. Deltoid Stretch
30 sec. per side

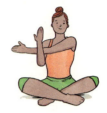

5. Wrist Flexion/ Extension
30 sec.

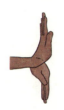

6. Wrist Rotations
30 sec.

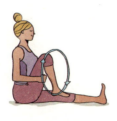

7. Seated Torso Circles
30 sec. each direction

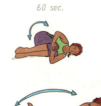

8. Easy Pose Side Bend
30 sec. each side

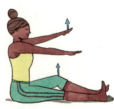

9. Revolved Easy Pose Salute Flow
30-60 sec., alternating sides

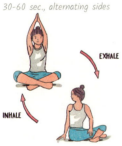

10. Seated Knee Rotations
30 sec. per side

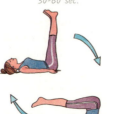

11. Cradle Pose
30 sec. per side

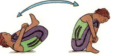

12. Staff Pose w/ Alternating Knee & Hand Lifts
30 sec.

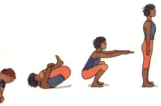

13. Boat to Half Boat Pose Flow
30-60 sec.

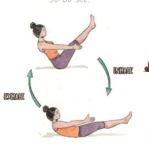

14. Half Plow Rollover Flow
30-60 sec.

15. Spinal Rock Pose
60 sec.

16. Wind Release to Mountain Pose Flow
30-60 sec.

Segment 2: Peak Flow

> Repeat poses 5-8 & 9-12, switching to the opposite side as necessary for asymmetrical poses.

1. Tree Pose
30 sec. per side

2. Upward Salute Side Bend
30 sec. per side

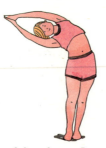

3. Chair Pose
30 sec.

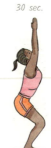

4. Forward Fold Flow
30 sec.

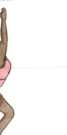

5. Downward Dog Crescent Lunge Flow
30-60 sec.

6. Low Lunge Pose w/ Cat-Cow
30 sec.

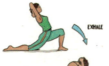

7. Crescent Low Lunge to Revolved Side Angle Pose Flow
30-60 sec.

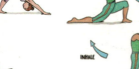

8. Vinyasa I
30 sec.

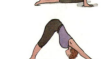

9. Downward Dog to Plank Pose Flow
30 sec.

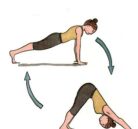

10. Three-Legged Downward Dog to Tiger Pose
30 sec.

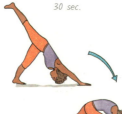
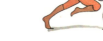

11. Pigeon Pose
30 sec.

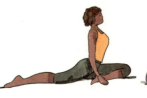

12. One-Legged King Pigeon Prep
30 sec.

13. Reverse Corpse Pose
30 sec.

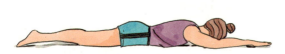

14. Prone to Supine Corpse Pose Flow
30-60 sec.

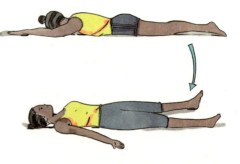

Segment 3: Cool Down

DATE

1. Wind Release Pose
60 sec.
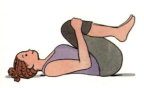

2. Happy Baby Pose
30–60 sec.
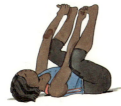

3. Supine Spinal Twist II Pose
30–60 sec. per side
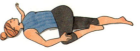

4. Fish Pose
60 sec.
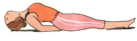

5. Full-Body Stretch Pose
30–60 sec.
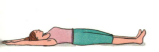

6. Half Plow Pose
30–60 sec.
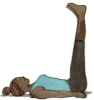

7. Sage Marichi Pose C
30 sec. per side
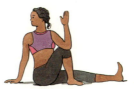

8. Sitting Swan Pose
30 sec. per side
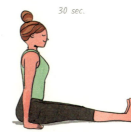

9. Upward-Facing Seated Straddle Pose
30–60 sec.
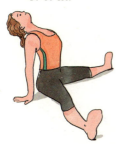

10. Seated Straddle Forward Fold Pose
30–60 sec.
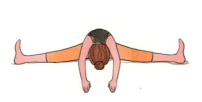

11. Staff Pose
30 sec.

12. Seated Forward Fold Pose
60 sec.
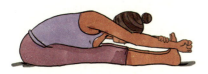

13. Corpse Pose
5 mins.
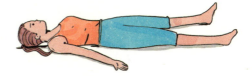

Food for Thought

Samadhi: the final limb of yoga.

The last limb of yoga, Samadhi, is a state of ecstasy, bliss, liberation from the external world, and union with the universe and the divine.

Similar to the final Kosha, Samadhi is meant to be experienced, rather than completed or obtained.

It's not a one-time feeling, but can only be sustained by consistent devotion to seeking it and developing your practice.

Just because you can't obtain this step and can simply experience doesn't make it any less of an important limb of Yoga, **so don't neglect it!**

Pranayama is the ultimate key to unlocking Samadhi and promoting inner awareness and growth.

Breathwork connects us to our mind, body, and soul, allows us to tap into the energies of our subtle bodies, and create awareness on and off the mat.

Keep working toward Samadhi through breath work, asanas, and meditation!

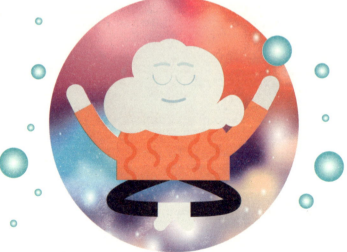

"Your life is a sacred transformation. It is about change, growth, discovery, movement, transformation, continuously expanding your vision of what is possible, stretching your learn, learning to see clearly and deeply, listening to your intuition, taking courage challenges at every step along the way." - Caroline Adams

Segment 1: Warm-Up

Full Session Exercise Guide:
habitnest.com/pages/yoga-day-61

1. Crocodile Pose

30 sec.

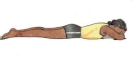

2. Locust to Wide-Legged Chariot Flow

60-90 sec.

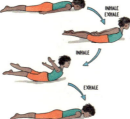

3. Prone to Supine Corpse Pose Flow

30 sec.

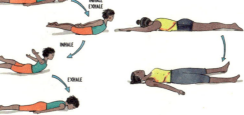

4. Half Plow Pose Flow

30-60 sec.

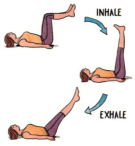

5. Bridge Pose Bound Angle Flow

60 sec., alternating legs

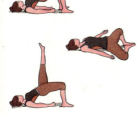

6. Full-Body Stretch to Seated Forward Fold Flow

30-60 sec.

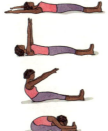

7. Wide-Legged Upward Plank

60 sec.

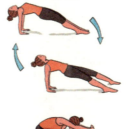

8. Boat to Half Boat Pose Flow

30-60 sec.

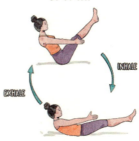

9. Rowing the Boat

30-60 sec.

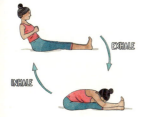

10. Garland Pose Salutation Flow

60 sec.

11. Woodchopper Pose Flow

30-60 sec.

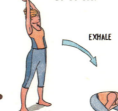

12. Wide-Legged Standing Backbend to Forward Fold Flow

60 sec.

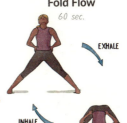

13. Dangling Intense Leg Stretch

60 sec.

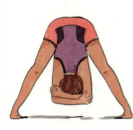

14. Intense Side Stretch Pose w/ Tiptoes

30 sec. per side

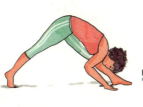

15. Moonflower/ Sunflower Pose Flow

30-60 sec.

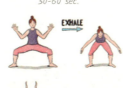
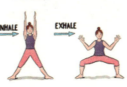

16. Volcano Pose

30-60 sec.

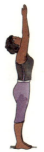

Segment 2: Peak Flow

Today, you'll be repeating the same Peak Flow you performed yesterday. This flow contains several moves that will help you in the process of advancing to more difficult poses.

> Repeat poses 5-8 & 9-12, switching to the opposite side as necessary for asymmetrical poses.

1. Tree Pose
30 sec. per side

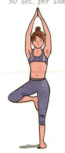

2. Upward Salute Side Bend
30 sec. per side

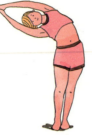

3. Chair Pose
30 sec.

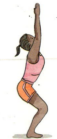

4. Forward Fold Flow
30 sec.

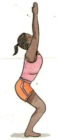

5. Downward Dog Crescent Lunge Flow
30-60 sec.

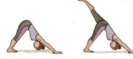

6. Low Lunge Pose w/ Cat-Cow
30 sec.

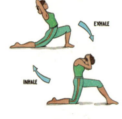

7. Crescent Low Lunge to Revolved Side Angle Pose Flow
30-60 sec.

8. Vinyasa I
30 sec.

9. Downward Dog to Plank Pose Flow
30 sec.

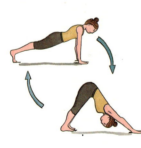

10. Three-Legged Downward Dog to Tiger Pose
30 sec.

11. Pigeon Pose
30 sec.

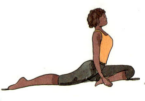

12. One-Legged King Pigeon Prep
30 sec.

13. Reverse Corpse Pose
30 sec.

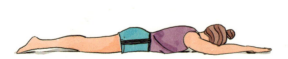

14. Prone to Supine Corpse Pose Flow
30-60 sec.

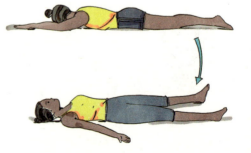

Segment 3: Cool Down

DATE

1. Rolling Happy Baby Variation Flow
60 sec.

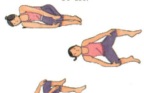

2. Bound Reclined Easy Pose
30-60 sec.

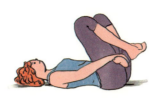

3. Half Plow Pose
30-60 sec.

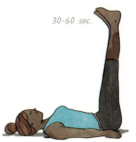

4. Supine Spinal Twist Pose
30 sec. per side

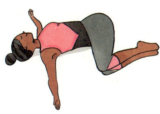

5. Seated Forward Fold Pose
30 sec.

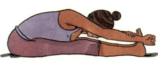

6. Half Happy Baby Pose
30 sec. per side

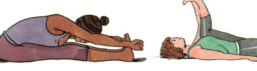

7. Sitting Swan Pose
30 sec. per side

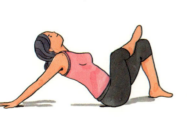

8. Half Cow Face Pose
30 sec. per side

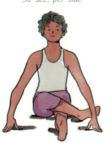

9. Half Cow Face Pose w/ Forward Fold
30 sec. per side

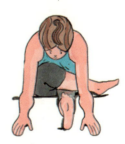

10. Full-Body Stretch Pose
30 sec.

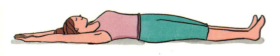

11. Corpse Pose
5 mins.

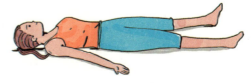

Food for Thought

Chakras: Third-Eye Chakra (Anja).

The sixth Chakra is the Third-Eye Chakra, located in the space between your eyebrows.

The Third Eye is said to be where our mind and body meet. It controls our **imagination, intuition, thinking patterns, decision-making process, and connection to a higher source** of knowledge.

A blockage of this Chakra can lead you to feel untrusting, close-minded, or lack intuitive guidance.

This Chakra is connected to:

- **Color** - Indigo/Purple
- **Element** - Light
- **Sound** - Om

You can foster a balance of this Chakra by:

- Practicing asanas that tap into this Chakra, such as Child's Pose, Plow Pose, or Downward Facing Dog.
- Incorporating Pranayama exercises that help to balance this Chakra, such as Alternate Nostril Breathing.
- Eating foods that nourish the Third-Eye, such as lavender teas, grapes, blueberries, or chocolate (yep, that's right, we said chocolate).

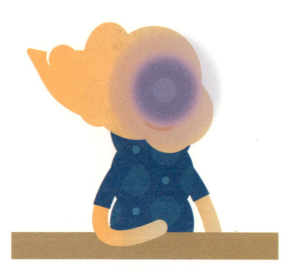

"Yoga is about clearing away whatever is in us that prevents our living in the most full and whole way. With yoga, we become aware of how and where we are restricted - in body, mind, and heart - and how gradually to open and release these blockages. As these blockages are cleared, our energy is freed. We start to feel more harmonious, more at one with ourselves. Our lives begin to flow - or we begin to flow more in our lives." -Cybele Tomlinson

Segment 1: Warm-Up

Full Session Exercise Guide:
habitnest.com/pages/yoga-day-62

1. Reclining Bound Angle Pose
60 sec.

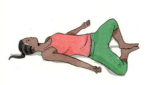

2. Revolved Abdomen Twist Pose
30 sec. per side

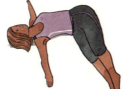

3. Forward-to-Backward Neck Stretch
30 sec., alternating

4. Side-to-Side Neck Stretches
30 sec. per side

5. Alternating Shoulder Shrugs
30 sec.

6. Seated Torso Circles
30 sec. each direction

7. Seated Forward Fold Prep
60 sec.

8. Seated Straddle Prep
60 sec.

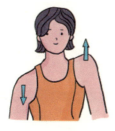
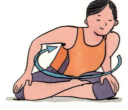
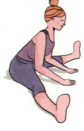
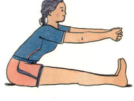

9. Sage Marichi Pose C
30 sec. per side

10. Seated Forward Fold Pose
60 sec.

11. Upward Facing Seated Straddle w/ Toe Grab
30-60 sec.

12. Cat-Cow Pose
30-60 sec., alternating

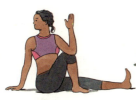
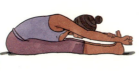
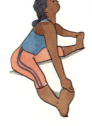
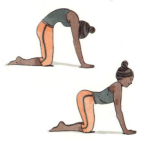

13. Table Top Side-to-Side Flow
30-60 sec., alternating sides

14. Balancing Table Top Knee-to-Nose Flow
30 sec. per side

15. Unilateral Balancing Table Top Pose
30 sec. per side

16. Wide Child's Pose
30-60 sec.

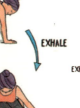
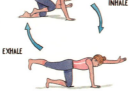
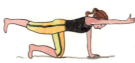
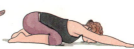

Segment 2: Peak Flow

> Repeat each pose in this segment, switching to the opposite side as necessary for asymmetrical poses.

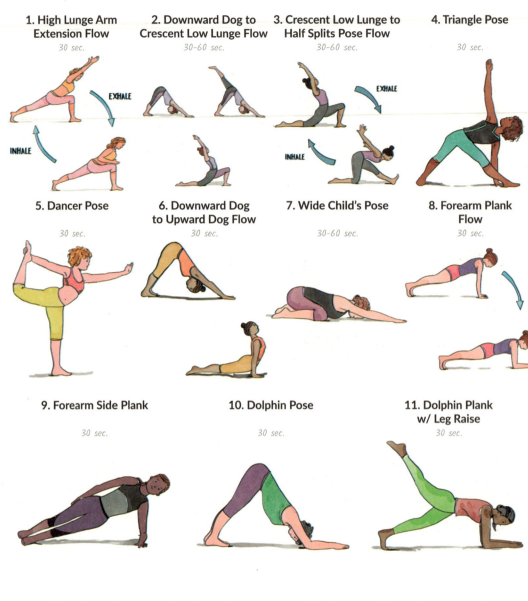

1. High Lunge Arm Extension Flow — 30 sec.
2. Downward Dog to Crescent Low Lunge Flow — 30-60 sec.
3. Crescent Low Lunge to Half Splits Pose Flow — 30-60 sec.
4. Triangle Pose — 30 sec.
5. Dancer Pose — 30 sec.
6. Downward Dog to Upward Dog Flow — 30 sec.
7. Wide Child's Pose — 30-60 sec.
8. Forearm Plank Flow — 30 sec.
9. Forearm Side Plank — 30 sec.
10. Dolphin Pose — 30 sec.
11. Dolphin Plank w/ Leg Raise — 30 sec.

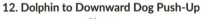

12. Dolphin to Downward Dog Push-Up — 30 sec.

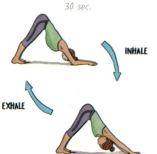

13. Downward Dog to Low Lunge Flow — 30-60 sec.

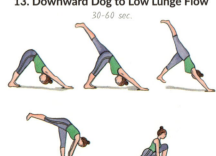

Segment 3: Cool Down

DATE

1. Child's Pose
30-60 sec.

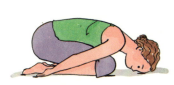

2. Cobra Pose
30-60 sec.

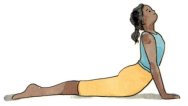

3. Plank Pose
30 sec.

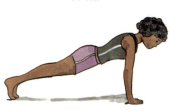

4. Downward-Facing Dog Pose
30 sec.

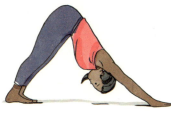

5. Table Top Pose
30 sec.

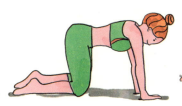

6. Puppy Dog Pose
30-60 sec.

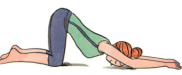

7. Puppy Dog Pose Neck Stretch
30 sec. per side

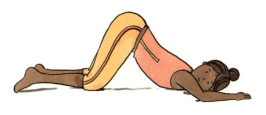

8. Revolved Puppy Dog Pose
30 sec. per side

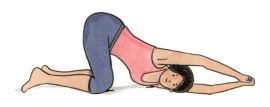

9. Half Wind Release Pose
30 sec. per side

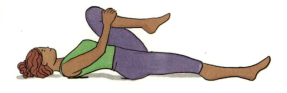

10. Corpse Pose
5 mins.

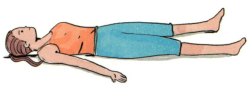

Food for Thought

Pratyahara: the link between yoga and your diet.

Even if you make the conscious decision to eat healthier, cleaner foods, that's not quite enough.

It's time to take a look at your eating habits.

- Start by **taking a long hard look at your current diet.** What food group do you eat way more than others? What foods are you overeating?

- **Create more variety in your diet.** Include plenty of leafy greens, veggies, healthy protein sources, and even healthy fats (like avocado)!

- **Stay hydrated throughout the day!** Being properly hydrated is absolutely necessary for proper mental and physical functioning.

- **Chew your food a lot and take it slow.** Swallowing food in a hurry makes it harder to digest. There's also a slight delay between your stomach becoming full and your brain receiving the signal to stop eating, so slowing down prevents you from overeating after your stomach is already satisfied.

- **Cook at home.** Limit the number of times you order out or eat at restaurants. Your health, waistline, and wallet will all thank you!

- **Eat breakfast in the mornings** to kickstart your digestion and control your appetite.

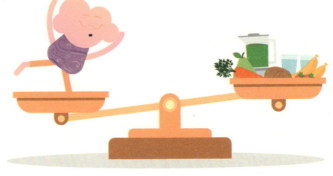

"True yoga is not about the shape of your body, but the shape of your life. Yoga is not to be performed; yoga is to be lived. Yoga doesn't care about what you have been; Yoga cares about the person you are becoming. Yoga is designed for a vast and profound purpose, and for it to be truly called yoga, its essence must be embodied." - Aadil Palkhivala

Segment 1: Warm-Up

Full Session Exercise Guide:
habitnest.com/pages/yoga-day-63

1. Crocodile Pose
30 sec.

2. Locust to Wide-Legged Chariot Flow
60-90 sec.

3. Prone to Supine Corpse Pose Flow
30 sec.

4. Half Plow Pose Flow
30-60 sec.

5. Bridge Pose Bound Angle Flow
60 sec., alternating legs

6. Full-Body Stretch to Seated Forward Fold Flow
30-60 sec.

7. Wide-Legged Upward Plank
60 sec.

8. Boat to Half Boat Pose Flow
30-60 sec.

9. Rowing the Boat
30-60 sec.

10. Garland Pose Salutation Flow
60 sec.

11. Woodchopper Pose Flow
30-60 sec.

12. Wide-Legged Standing Backbend to Forward Fold Flow
60 sec.

13. Dangling Intense Leg Stretch
60 sec.

14. Intense Side Stretch Pose w/ Tiptoes
30 sec. per side

15. Moonflower/Sunflower Pose Flow
30-60 sec.

16. Volcano Pose
30-60 sec.

Segment 2: Peak Flow

> Repeat poses 1-12, switching to the opposite side as necessary for asymmetrical poses.

1. Chair Pose
30 sec.

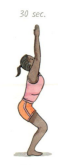

2. Straight-Legged Warrior I Salute Flow
30 sec.

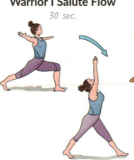

3. Warrior II Intense Leg Stretch Flow
60 sec.

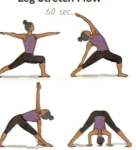

4. Revolved Wide-Legged Forward Fold Pose
30-60 sec.

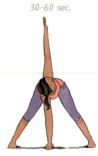

5. Goddess Pose
30-45 sec.

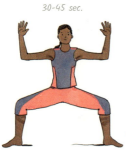

6. Warrior II Pose
30 sec.

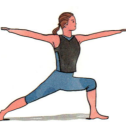

7. Reverse Warrior Pose
30 sec.

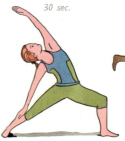

8. Warrior III Pose
30 sec.

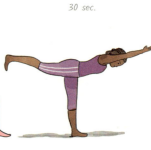

9. Sugarcane Pose
30 sec.

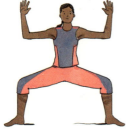

10. Half Moon Pose
30 sec.

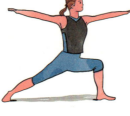

11. Dancer Pose
30 sec.

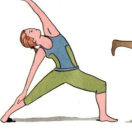

12. Standing Forward Fold Pose
30 sec.

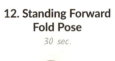

13. Garland Pose
30 sec.

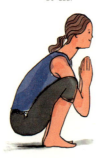

14. Bound Angle Pose
60 sec.

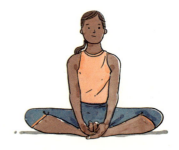

Segment 3: Cool Down

DATE

1. Seated Star Pose
60 sec.

2. Head-to-Knee Pose
30 sec. per side

3. Boat Pose w/ Knees Bent
30 sec.

4. Easy Boat Pose
30-60 sec.

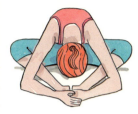
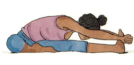
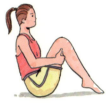
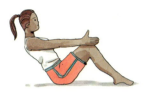

5. Staff Pose w/ Hands Back
30 sec.

6. Reverse Table Top Pose
30 sec.

7. Caterpillar Pose
30-60 sec.

8. Supine Knee Circles
30-60 sec.

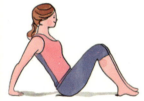
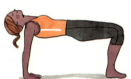
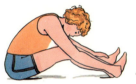
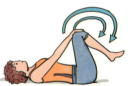

9. Half Wind Release Leg Raise Flow
30 sec. per side

10. Supine Spinal Twist II Pose
30 sec. per side

11. Supine Tree Pose
30 sec. per side

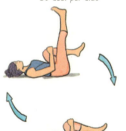
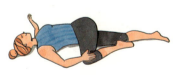
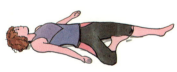

12. Full-Body Stretch w/ Gesture of the Pond
30-60 sec.

13. Corpse Pose
5 mins.

INHALE

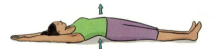

EXHALE

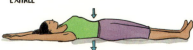
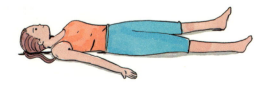

Food for Thought

Chakras: Crown Chakra (Sahasrara).

The final Chakra is the Crown Chakra, appropriately located at the very top of your head. This Chakra has to do with our inner beauty and our connection to the spiritual world.

It goes beyond the physical experience of being human, focusing on the spiritual aspects and, ultimately, enlightenment.

The properties of this Chakra are:

- **Color** - Violet or White
- **Element** - Cosmic Energy
- **Sound** - Om
  (same as Third-Eye Chakra)

A blocked Crown Chakra can lead to a lack of focus, confusion, lost connection to the spiritual world, and poor physical functioning.

You can bring balance to this Chakra through asanas and breathwork exercises that tap into the Crown Chakra (such as Child's Pose and Alternate Nostril Breathing).

Aim to keep this Chakra open and balanced so as not to disrupt the spiritual aspect of your yoga practice!

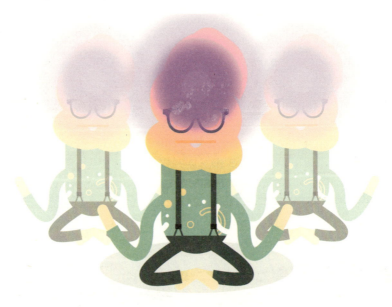

"You are not a drop in the ocean. You are the entire ocean in a drop." - Rumi

Segment 1: Warm-Up

Full Session Exercise Guide:
habitnest.com/pages/yoga-day-64

1. Crocodile Pose
30 sec.

2. Locust to Wide-Legged Chariot Flow
60-90 sec.

3. Prone to Supine Corpse Pose Flow
30 sec.

4. Half Plow Pose Flow
30-60 sec.

5. Bridge Pose Bound Angle Flow
60 sec., alternating legs

6. Full-Body Stretch to Seated Forward Fold Flow
30-60 sec.

7. Wide-Legged Upward Plank
60 sec.

8. Boat to Half Boat Pose Flow
30-60 sec.

9. Rowing the Boat
30-60 sec.

10. Garland Pose Salutation Flow
60 sec.

11. Woodchopper Pose Flow
30-60 sec.

12. Wide-Legged Standing Backbend to Forward Fold Flow
60 sec.

13. Dangling Intense Leg Stretch
60 sec.

14. Intense Side Stretch Pose w/ Tiptoes
30 sec. per side

15. Moonflower/Sunflower Pose Flow
30-60 sec.

16. Volcano Pose
30-60 sec.

Segment 2: Peak Flow

> Repeat poses 1-4 & 5-8, switching to the opposite side as necessary for asymmetrical poses.

1. Tree Pose
30-60 sec.

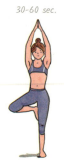

2. Tree Pose w/ Side Bends
30 sec.

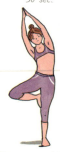

3. Chair Pose
30 sec.

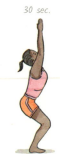

4. Revolved Chair Pose
30 sec.

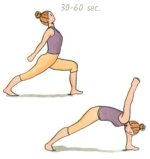

5. Downward Dog to Upward Dog Pose Flow
30-60 sec.

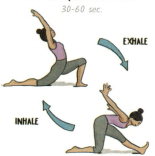

6. Three-Legged Downward-Facing Dog Pose
30-60 sec.

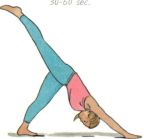

7. Bound Warrior to Humble Warrior Pose Flow
30-60 sec.

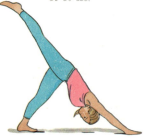

8. Crescent Low Lunge to Half Split Pose Flow
30-60 sec.

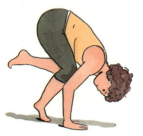

9. Crow Pose w/ Toe Taps
30 sec. per side

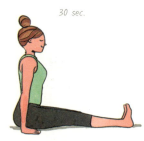

10. Staff Pose
30 sec.

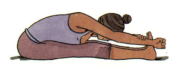

11. Seated Forward Fold Pose
60 sec.

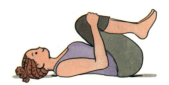

12. Wind Release Pose
60 sec.

Segment 3: Cool Down

DATE

1. Fish Pose
60 sec.

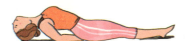

2. Full-Body Stretch Pose
60 sec.

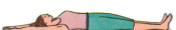

3. Half Wind Release Pose
30 sec. per side

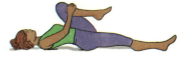

4. Wind Release Pose
60 sec.

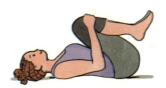

5. Scorpion Twist Pose
30 sec. per side

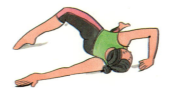

6. Supine Butterfly Pose Wings
30-60 sec.

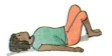

7. Supine Windshield Wipers
30 sec. per side

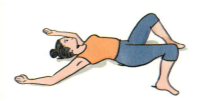

8. Reverse Pigeon Pose
30 sec. per side

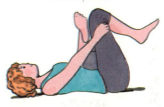

9. Reclined Half Cow Face Pose
30-60 sec. per side

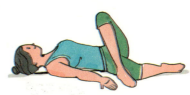

10. Reclined Cow Face Pose
30 sec., then reverse legs & repeat

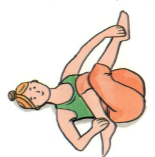

11. Corpse Pose
5 mins.

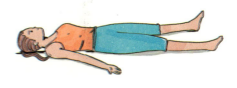

Favorite Resources

Asanas: try YogaGlo.

Glo is a platform that offers over 3,000 yoga videos that focus on 12 different styles of yoga, along with meditations and in-depth explorations of the ancient Yogic teachings and sacred texts.

Their classes range from beginner to advanced, with plenty of options available for students of all levels. It even includes partner practices, prenatal yoga, and post-natal workouts that include the whole family.

Whatever your current abilities and goals, Glo has something for you! There are many different teachers, all with their own styles, so you're bound to find a teacher you like.

Glo offers affordable monthly and annual subscription options that allow you unlimited access to their full library of pre-recorded classes, as well as scheduled live classes!

Give it a shot by visiting: www.glo.com! It's an amazing resource for keeping your practice going strong long after you've completed your habit journey.

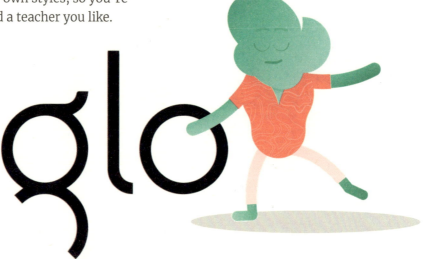

"The beautiful thing about yoga is that there are so many different approaches. As we go through our life cycles, hopefully, we are able to find a practice that suits us." - Tiffany Cruikshank

Segment 1: Warm-Up

Full Session Exercise Guide:
habitnest.com/pages/yoga-day-65

1. Alternate Nostril Breathing
2-4 mins.

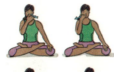
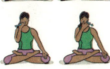

2. Alternating Shoulder Shrugs
30 sec.

3. Alternating Elbow Flapping
30 sec.

4. Deltoid Stretch
30 sec. per side

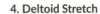

5. Wrist Flexion/Extension
30 sec.

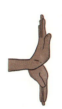

6. Wrist Rotations
30 sec.

7. Seated Torso Circles
30 sec. each direction

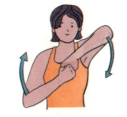

8. Easy Pose Side Bend
30 sec. each side

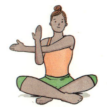

9. Revolved Easy Pose Salute Flow
30-60 sec., alternating sides

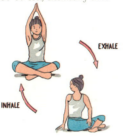

10. Seated Knee Rotations
30 sec. per side

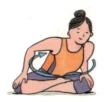

11. Cradle Pose
30 sec. per side

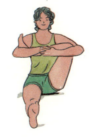

12. Staff Pose w/ Alternating Knee & Hand Lifts
30 sec.

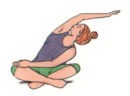

13. Boat to Half Boat Pose Flow
30-60 sec.

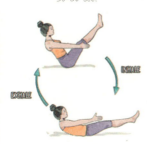

14. Half Plow Rollover Flow
30-60 sec.

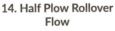
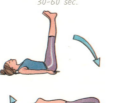

15. Spinal Rock Pose
60 sec.

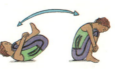

16. Wind Release to Mountain Pose Flow
30-60 sec.

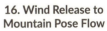
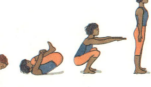

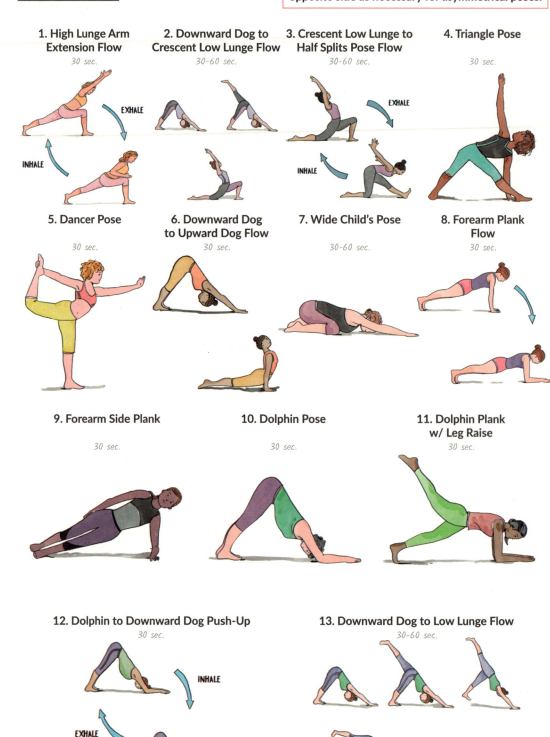

Segment 3: Cool Down

DATE

1. Thunderbolt Pose w/ Cat-Cow
30 sec.

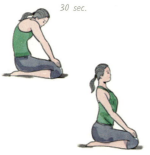

2. Revolved Thunderbolt Pose
30 sec. per side

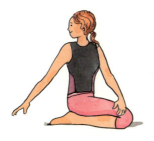

3. Thunderbolt Pose Salute
60 sec.

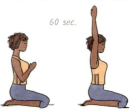

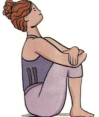

4. Puppy Dog Pose
30-60 sec.

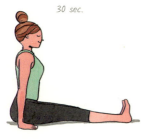

5. Resting Half Frog Pose
30 sec. per side

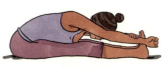

6. Seated Wind Release Pose
30-60 sec.

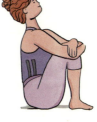

7. Staff Pose
30 sec.

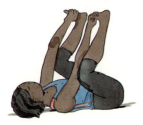

8. Seated Forward Fold Pose
60 sec.

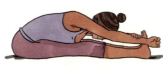

9. Sitting Swan Pose
30 sec. per side

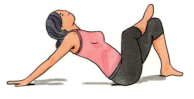

10. Happy Baby Pose
30-60 sec.

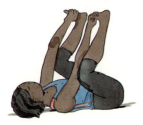

11. Reclining Bound Angle Pose
30-60 sec.

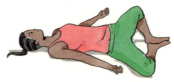

12. Corpse Pose
5 mins.

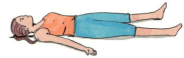

Flow 66

Congratulations!!!

YOU DID IT!!! You're absolutely amazing, and you deserve a huuuuge pat on the back!

You made it through 66 days of building and strengthening your personal yoga practice, which is an incredible feat.

To top it off, you now have a connection to this valuable habit that is absolutely unbreakable. You can tap into the skills you have learned along the way any time you need them.

Don't let your journey stop here, though! Whether you continue building upon your yoga practice, or you try to build a completely new habit, never stop chasing personal growth! We're here for you, no matter what path you choose from here!

Much love and appreciation from the entire Habit Nest team. Thank you for being the amazing person you are, and we hope to continue walking this path with you!

Note: We LOVE sharing stories of our users and what their lives looked like BEFORE using the journal compared to where they are NOW!

If you want to share your story with us, you can do so here:

habitnest.com/yogatestimonial

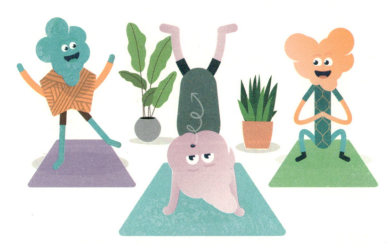

"Notice the silence. Notice your heart. Still beating. Still fighting. You made it after all. You made it another day. And you can make it one more. You're doing just fine." - Charlotte Eriksson

Segment 1: Warm-Up

Full Session Exercise Guide:
habitnest.com/pages/yoga-day-66

1. Seated Torso Circles
30 sec. each direction

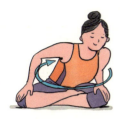

2. Shoulder Socket Rotations
30-60 sec.

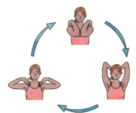

3. Revolved Easy Pose Salute Flow
60 sec., alternating sides

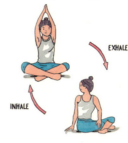

4. Easy Pose Side Bend
30 sec. per side

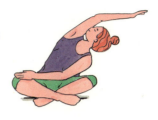

5. Seated Butterfly Pose Wings
30 sec.

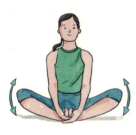

6. Bound Butterfly Wings Flow
30-60 sec.

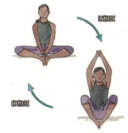

7. Fish Pose w/ Butterfly Legs
60 sec.

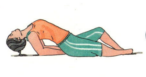

8. Seated Star Pose
60 sec.

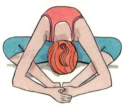

9. Table Top Pose
30 sec.

10. Table Top Pose Wrist Stretch
30 sec.

11. Cat-Cow Rib Circles
30-45 sec. each direction

12. Plank Knee-to-Nose Flow
30 sec. per side

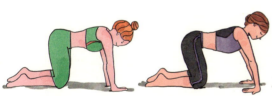
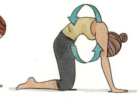
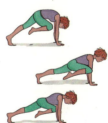
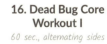
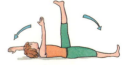

13. Reclined Single Hip Rotation
30 sec. per side

14. Wind Release Flow
30-60 sec.

15. Half Plow Pose Leg Flow
60 sec.

16. Dead Bug Core Workout I
60 sec., alternating sides

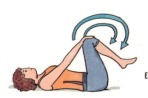
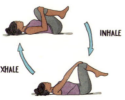
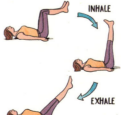
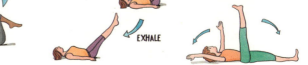

Segment 2: Peak Flow

Repeat each pose in this segment, switching to the opposite side as necessary for asymmetrical poses.

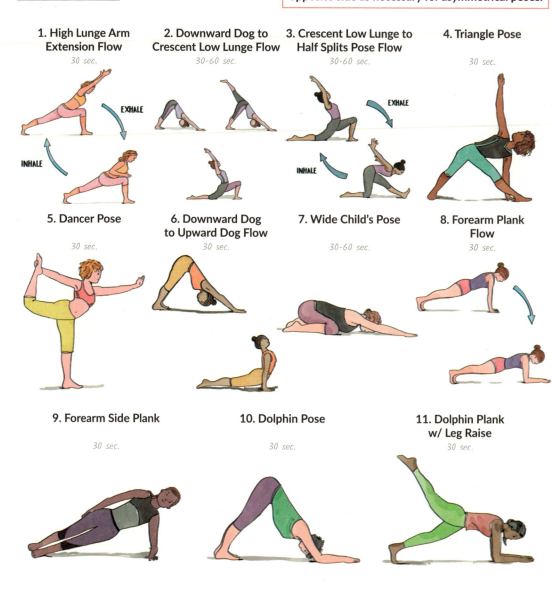

1. High Lunge Arm Extension Flow — 30 sec.
2. Downward Dog to Crescent Low Lunge Flow — 30-60 sec.
3. Crescent Low Lunge to Half Splits Pose Flow — 30-60 sec.
4. Triangle Pose — 30 sec.
5. Dancer Pose — 30 sec.
6. Downward Dog to Upward Dog Flow — 30 sec.
7. Wide Child's Pose — 30-60 sec.
8. Forearm Plank Flow — 30 sec.
9. Forearm Side Plank — 30 sec.
10. Dolphin Pose — 30 sec.
11. Dolphin Plank w/ Leg Raise — 30 sec.

12. Dolphin to Downward Dog Push-Up — 30 sec.

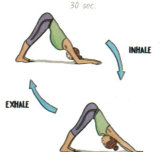

13. Downward Dog to Low Lunge Flow — 30-60 sec.

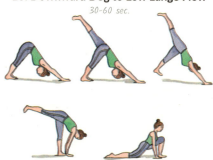

Segment 3: Cool Down

DATE

1. Locust to Wide-Legged Chariot Flow
60-90 sec.

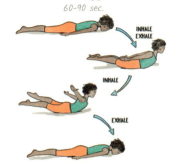

2. Crocodile Pose
30 sec.

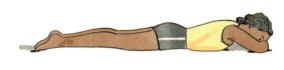

3. Downward-Facing Dog Pose
30 sec.

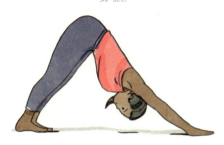

4. Sleeping Swan Pose
30-60 sec. per side

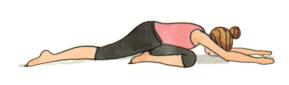

5. Thread the Needle Pose
30 sec. per side

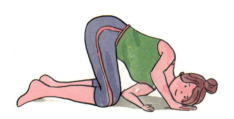

6. Reclined Leg Stretch Flow
60 sec.

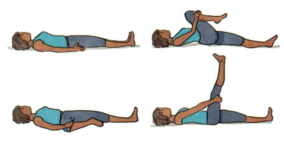

7. Full-Body Stretch to Wind Release Flow
30 sec.

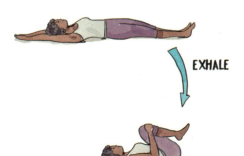

8. Corpse Pose
5 mins.

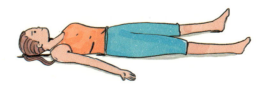

Recap Questions

1. What did my life look like before I began this practice? What is different, and how do I feel now compared to then?

2. What unexpected benefits in my life (on and off the mat) and well-being did I gain by consistently building my practice?

3. What is my relationship and inner dialogue with myself like now compared to when I began? Do I love, understand, and appreciate myself more now?

4. What elements of my practice need to be changed or adjusted to ensure that I stick with it moving forward? How can I address them?

5. What kind of tracking or accountability methods can I use to stay consistent moving forward?

6. What key factors do I want to remember in the future to guide me if I fall off track? What can I do to ensure that I get back on track?

Congratulations!

You've mastered the Yoga Sidekick Journal!

Phase 3 Done.

- Fin -

So... What Now?

Although you should feel very accomplished for getting through this entire journal... know that you built this habit to continually improve your life. Don't stop now. This is only the beginning.

One huge factor to this is tracking your progress.

Once you stop tracking, it makes it exponentially easier for you to lose your momentum in your daily yoga practice (due to the lack of accountability with yourself).

Remember: **Every day that you commit to your yoga practice and apply principles of yoga in your life, you will continue to learn and grow into the best version of yourself.**

You only stand to gain from continuing with your yoga practice.

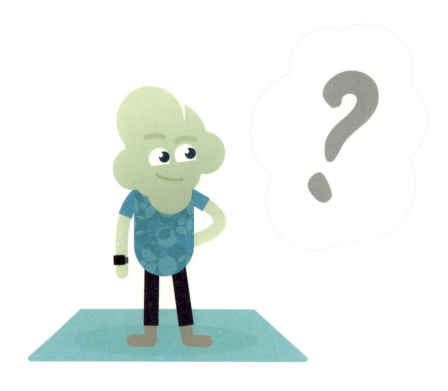

Shop Habit Nest Products

Lifestyle Products

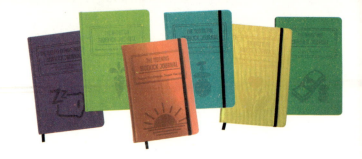

All of our lifestyle journals come with **daily content** (including Pro-Tips, Daily Challenges, Practical Resources, & more) to inspire you and give you bite-sized information to use along your journey. They also contain **daily questions aimed at holding you accountable** to ingraining that habit into your life.

The Morning Sidekick Journal Series

A set of guided morning planners that help you conquer your mornings and conquer your life. This complete 4-volume series covers one year of morning routines.

The Evening Routine & Sleep Sidekick Journal

Helps you to wind down your days peacefully, prepare for each next day, and get the most rejuvenating sleep of your life.

The Gratitude Sidekick Journal Series

A set of research-based journals that will help make an attitude of appreciation a core part of who you are. There are 3 Volumes in total.

The Meditation Sidekick Journal

Built to give you all the tools you need to stay consistent with a meditation practice.

The Nutrition Sidekick Journal

Your nutrition tracker, informational guide, and coach, all in one.

The Budgeting Sidekick Journal Series

The most simple-yet-effective budgeting guide in the world, helping you find full clarity on your budgeting goals and to achieve financial freedom. Set spending goals, track your daily spending, and reconcile along the way. Contains two volumes, which cover well over a year of budgeting.

Fitness Products

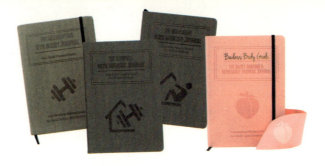

Our no-nonsense fitness books have fully guided fitness routines. No thinking required; just open the books and follow along.

The Weightlifting Gym Buddy Journal Series

A set of guided personal training programs aimed at helping you have the best workouts of your life. This complete 4-volume series covers one year of weightlifting workouts.

The Bodyweight / Dumbbell Home Workout Journals

Specifically focus on HOME workout programs that require minimal-to-no equipment to complete.

The Badass Body Goals Journal

An at-home-friendly fitness journal that focuses on HIIT and circuit workouts. This journal comes with a full video guide you can play and follow along.

Other Products

The Habit Nest Daily Planner

Plan your day including your top priorities, smaller 5-minute tasks, and all your to-dos. Get optional suggestions for ways to start your mornings and end your evenings with as well.

George The Short-Necked Giraffe (Children's Book)

Follow along George's journey as he learns the hard way that fully accepting himself, exactly the way he is, is the only path to living his happiest life.

Shop all products here: **habitnest.com/store**

The Habit Nest Mobile App

The Habit Nest app offers a **digital representation of our journals**, with the benefit of improved tracking, varying ways to showcase content, and gamification, and more.

When Habit Nest was initially founded, it was supposed to be in mobile app form from the start.

As a team of three young founders with no outside funding to get a mobile app built, we started with paper journals that worked using the same concept, which you're currently holding.

5 years and hundreds of thousands of journals sold later, we were finally able to create our mobile app and released it at the end of 2021.

We will always continue to print physical journals for every habit we release, only now, they'll also be put into the app so that everyone can experience our habit journeys in the way that suits them best.

If you're interested in seeing seeing whether the app is right for you, feel free to see more at **habitnest.com/app**

With a lot of love,

Mikey Ahdoot, Ari Banayan, & Amir Atighehchi
Co-Founders of Habit Nest

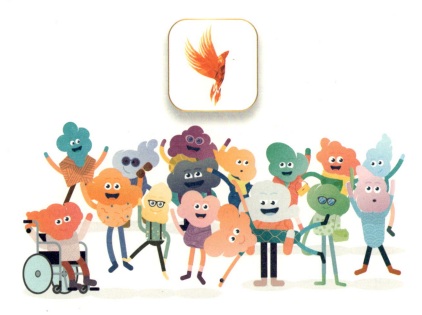

The Phoenixes Access Pass

We released *The Phoenixes* – Habit Nest's Special Access Pass – in 2022.

Anyone who purchases a Phoenix gets:

1. **Lifetime access** to the Habit Nest app.

2. Access to a **Learn2Earn system** we're building within the app, in which you will have chances to earn prizes/rewards for using our app to build better habits.

3. **First dibs** on new journal releases & our best discounts.

If you're interested in purchasing a Phoenix, visit:

https://habitnest.com/vip

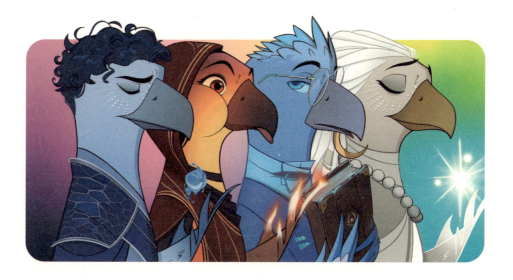

For more information, follow The Phoenixes on Twitter: **@thephoenixesnft**